YOGA SECRETS
FOR
BUSINESS
SUCCESS

**TRANSITION STRESS MANAGEMENT
IN THE 21ST CENTURY**

YOGA SECRETS FOR BUSINESS SUCCESS

TRANSITION STRESS MANAGEMENT IN THE 21ST CENTURY

BY

DARSHAN SINGH KHALSA

THE LYONS PRESS

GUILFORD, CONNECTICUT
An Imprint of The Globe Pequot Press

Always consult your physician before beginning this or any other exercise program. Nothing in this manual is to be construed as medical advice. The benefits attributed to the practice of Kundalini Yoga come from centuries-old yogic tradition. Results will vary with individuals.

The Lyons Press is an imprint of the Globe Pequot Press
First Lyons Press edition, April 2002
Printed in Korea
ISBN 1-58574-518-9

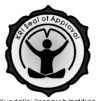

Kundalini Research Institute

This Seal of Approval is granted only to those products which have been approved through the KRI Review process for accuracy and integrity of those portions which embody the technology of Kundalini Yoga and 3HO Lifestyle as taught by Yogi Bhajan.

TABLE OF CONTENTS

BELONGING

SELF-ESTEEM

SELF-REALIZATION

APPENDICES

DEDICATION

This work is dedicated to my teacher

Siri Singh Sahib Bhai Sahib Harbhajan
Singh Khalsa Yogi Ji,
also known as

Yogi Bhajan
Master of Kundalini Yoga

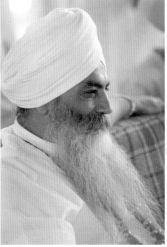

who graciously brought the
technology of Kundalini Yoga
to the Western world
and inspired generations to
reach their
highest human potential.

May all those who come in contact with these
teachings be blessed to practice them purely
and to KEEP UP !

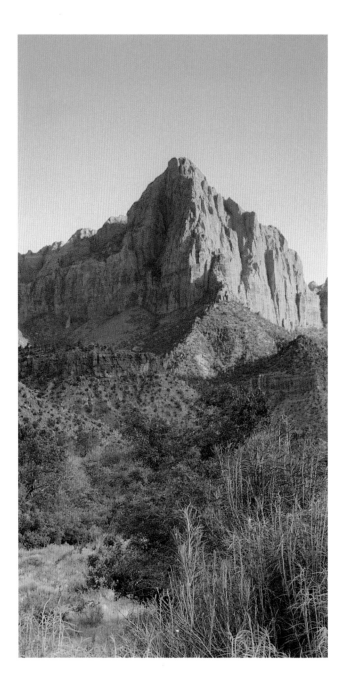

ACKNOWLEDGMENTS

This work is reaching a wider audience through the professionalism and inspiration of agent Sarah Piel of Arthur Pine Associates and editor Ann Treistman of The Lyons Press. Thanks to the efforts of The Lyons Press design team, the illustrations are in color and the book lays flat so you can really make use of it. Thank you for your labors of love.

My thanks to Brad Harper, Bruce Grant, Guru Amrit Kaur Khalsa, Guru Roop Kaur Khalsa, Dr. Hari Simran Singh Khalsa, Jim Norman, Jiwan Shakti Singh Boll, Dr. Jodha Singh Khalsa, John O'Connor, Sewa Singh Khalsa, Siri Ram Kaur Khalsa, and William and Ruth Freedman for inspiration and support of Transition Stress Management and this project in particular.

For manuscript editorial assistance and for ensuring accuracy of the yoga technology, I am indebted to Guru Roop Kaur Khalsa, Guru Simran Kaur Khalsa, Satya Kaur Khalsa of KRI, Shakti Parwha Kaur Khalsa, and William Freedman.

For sage advice in entering the world of publishing, I am indebted to Dr. Dharma Singh Khalsa, Lynella Grant, Shakta Kaur Khalsa, and Shakti Parwha Kaur Khalsa.

I am grateful to Atma Kaur Khalsa, Bibi Bhani Kaur Khalsa, Guru Bachan Kaur Khalsa, Guru Kar Singh Khalsa, Guru Simran Kaur Khalsa, Livtar Singh Khalsa, Ravi Nam Kaur Khalsa, and Sat Jivan Singh Khalsa for catching the vision early on.

Thanks to Chris Bassett and Margaret Makie for photographic studio assistance, and to yoga models Angela Belote, Ben Bowen, Jeff Bade, Jessica Ruiz, Sat Rattan Kaur Khalsa, and Sat Siri Kaur Khalsa.

I am grateful to my wife Akal Kaur Khalsa for her encouragement and support.

INTRODUCTION

I worked for over twenty-two years in management in the corporate environment, having joined a very small computer reseller start-up company at the beginning of the microcomputer revolution. The company eventually grew to become a multibillion dollar Fortune 500 computer distributor and systems integrator. It was a high-tech, high-stress environment. I found the work exciting but, as in any company, there were daily challenges, deadlines, pressures, and of course, office politics. These stressful challenges posed not only a threat to my abil-

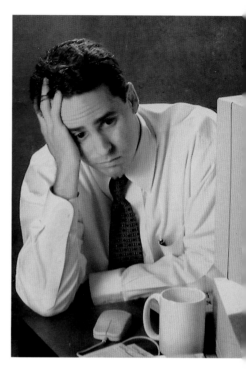

ity to excel, but their cumulative effect could have led to physical, emotional, and mental breakdown.

To thrive and succeed in the business world, many self-management skills are necessary, including the abilities to manage stress, relax quickly at will, energize when necessary, handle sleep deprivation, relieve headaches, overcome fear and depression, manage anger, sharpen concentration, expand intuition, experience tranquility, relieve grumpiness, persevere to completion, substitute good habits for bad, improve decision making, improve self-esteem and personal magnetism, and manifest your potential.

This book shows you how to develop these abilities through short and simple exercises with proven results for the busy working person. I have successfully used these techniques for nearly three decades to manage stress, be more productive, deal with negative emotions, and improve many other aspects of life in the work environment. Some exercises can be practiced right at your desk at work whenever you have a few minutes available. Other exercises can be practiced at home.

If you practice any of the techniques in this book, your life will be better. But don't take my word for it. Try these simple and effective but little-known techniques, and you will see the results.

They work because they are based on the ancient teachings of Kundalini Yoga. Yoga has been practiced for thousands of years by millions of people. Anyone can practice these techniques to reduce stress and improve self control. Yoga is a science because the results are known; it is an art in the way you practice and apply the technology to your life.

Yogi Bhajan says that as we expand our awareness through the practice of yoga, we evolve from individual consciousness to group consciousness, and from group consciousness to universal consciousness.

We have two selves: the known self, and the unknown potential Self. The goal of yoga is for each person to experience their unknown potential Self. The yoga exercises and meditations in the chapters of this book have been sequenced in ascending priority from those that focus on personal self (physical survival and mental/emotional security), through interacting with others (longing to belong and self-esteem), to connecting with our unknown potential Self (self-realization). The sequence is similar to Maslow's

SELF
ESTEEM
BELONGING
SECURITY
SURVIVAL

Hierarchy of Needs.[1] In the table of contents of this book you will see section headers for the evolving priorities of the Expansion of Consciousness: survival, security, belonging, self-esteem, self-realization.

Pick a chapter whose title strikes a chord within you, read the chapter, and practice the technique. Through the blessings of my teacher Yogi Bhajan, and his guru, Guru Ram Das, you are bound to have a better life.

What Is Yoga?

Yoga is a science of the mind, an ancient system of exercise that includes thousands of physical and mental exercises designed to strengthen and balance the body, rejuvenate the nervous system, and concentrate the mind. Yoga integrates body and mind so that you can experience your essence: inner peace.

Yoga is not a religion; it is a technology and a discipline similar to martial arts. You can be of any faith or religion, or none, and still gain the healing benefits of yoga.

Yoga is a superb stress-management technology and a means of achieving personal excellence. Today yoga is widely used for many purposes. International competitive swimming teams use yogic breathing techniques to efficiently fill their lungs with oxygen before they swim. Popular singers and actors use yogic techniques to enhance their physical performance and to combat the fatigue of exhaustive work schedules.

Yoga was originally developed as a way to enhance self-knowledge. The practice of yoga integrates body and mind in order to achieve and maintain a higher consciousness. The word yoga, like the English word "yoke," has the same origin in the Sanskrit word *yugit*, which means to link together. To achieve this linking together, yoga employs a number of very powerful tools: physical practice, various body pos-

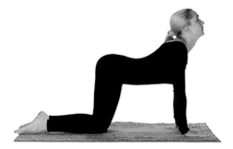

tures, breathing techniques, mental concentration, and meditation. One of the central aspects of yoga is that you yourself should be able to control your life. The techniques provided in this book can help you do so.

What Is Kundalini Yoga?

Kundalini Yoga, the yoga of awareness, is a comprehensive and effective form of yoga that can be practiced by everyone. It is an ideal practice for people with busy lifestyles because they can experience an immediate and direct effect in the shortest amount of time. In fact, most Kundalini Yoga exercises are practiced for no more than three minutes at a time, usually followed by a short relaxation.

Kundalini Yoga is so effective because each exercise typically combines several factors: certain physical postures that strengthen the body, plus specific breathing techniques and meditation designed to strengthen the nervous system, stimulate the glandular system, concentrate the mind, and energize the body while also relaxing it. It keeps the body in shape and trains the mind to be strong and flexible in the face of stress and change. As one advances in years, yoga keeps the body healthy and the mind clear.

Kundalini Yoga is a comprehensive discipline that includes all forms of yoga within it, although it is not the kind of yoga one usually sees on television. Because Kundalini Yoga is effective and precise in its effects, it must be taught by a qualified teacher. Until little more than thirty years ago, Kundalini Yoga was virtually unknown in the western hemisphere because it had remained a well-kept secret in the Himalayas for thousands of years. We are fortunate in that Yogi Bhajan, Master of Kundalini Yoga, relocated from India to the United States more than thirty years ago and trained thousands of teachers over the years.

Kundalini Yoga is not just a small thing and neither is it a big thing. It is *the* thing. And man shall need it. And it shall be needed by men just to survive. It will be an essential part of life, because there will be no time and then in a few minutes men shall and women shall have the capacity to renew themselves. It will give them the reorganization, reconciliation, and give them the resurrection they need to come out of whatever deep depression and cold depression they shall be in . . . . There once was a time the reach of a man was only twelve miles. Today the whole planet earth is just one game. So please qualify yourself, and whatever *yoga kriya* [exercise set] suits you personally, you can practice it in daily life, so that you can always bring your balance and your excellence.[2]

—Yogi Bhajan

How Kundalini Yoga Works

You already have all the equipment necessary to do yoga. You have the body, spine, nervous system, endocrine glands, lungs and breath, circulatory system, brain, and so on. According to the yogis, the *kundalini* energy—the energy to experience your unknown potential and infinite self—is stored at the base of the spine. The word *kundalini* comes from the word *kundal*, which means the curl of the hair of the beloved. Thus the *kundalini* energy is coiled and stored at the base of the spine waiting to be activated.

Through the practice of yoga, the body gradually becomes healthier and the nervous system stronger, and the mind develops the ability to concentrate. Based upon that platform, through various exercises combined with powerful breathing, yogis draw *prana*, the life energy of the universe, into the body and store it from the eighth vertebra on down. Then through other exercises where the various locks such as Root Lock, Diaphragm Lock and Neck Lock are applied, they apply pressure to raise this energy up the central channel of the spine to the higher brain centers, to stimulate the pituitary gland (the seat of intuition) and the pineal gland (the seat of universal consciousness). Once the *kundalini* rises, you become superconscious and the wisest of the wise. You can know your total surroundings and live as a blessed being. It is a matter of practical experience.

The practice of Kundalini Yoga directly affects the nervous system, and stimulates the endocrine gland system. Each of the endocrine glands plays a major role in the body's functioning. The following is a brief summary of their major effects: The gonad secretions affect your potency and creativity as well as the ability to sit still for meditation; the adrenals affect energy level and stress reaction; the pancreas affects blood sugar and digestion; the thymus affects the immune system; the parathyroids and thyroid regulate body metabolism, health, and the aging process; the pituitary regulates all the other endocrine glands and affects intuition; the pineal gland regulates sleep cycles and affects higher states of consciousness.

Each Kundalini Yoga exercise typically has posture, breathing, mantra, and movement; therefore, through the combination of all these factors, it gets results faster than other kinds of yoga. Basic postures are discussed below, and the kriyas that follow in this book combine postures with movement. Breathing is covered in the Breath to the Rescue chapter. A mantra is composed of scientific sounds derived from the ancient Sanskrit language that does to us what it means, unlike English. In English, the integration of sound and meaning is rare; it is known as onomatopoeia, the use of words whose sound suggests the sense. The healing power of this kind of sound is very powerful.

For example, when you create and extend the sound "maaaaaaaaah," you can feel it open up the heart center. Imagine an entire language in which each sound and word, their meanings, and their psycho-physiological effects upon both the speaker and listener are all completely consistent. That is the power of Sanskrit and its daughter languages, which are the primary languages of mantras. There are no secret mantras in Kundalini Yoga. A summary of the mantras presented in this book can be found in the Appendices (page 181).

BASIC POSTURES
EASY POSE

Most of the meditations in this book require you to sit with your spine straight and your posture balanced. The ideal sitting posture (asana) *is Easy Pose, a comfortable crossl-egged sitting position, sitting up straight with the spinal vertebrae aligned like a perfect stack of coins (see Fig. Intro-1).*

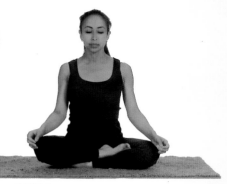

INTRO 1

To get into Easy Pose: Sit with the legs out straight. Pull the left foot in to the groin. Place the right foot over the ankle of the left foot so that it rests near the thigh. Straighten the spine. The feet can be arranged in either order.

The feet should be bare when practicing yoga to enhance energy flow throughout the body, unless you are practicing yoga at your workstation or some other place where being barefoot is not possible.

When you sit for meditation it is important that you feel balanced and stable. If you meditate in an off-balance posture, you run the risk of mis-directing the energy and blood circulation that is stimulated by the exercise. Your posture should always feel well balanced and comfortable to you, and should be balanced in such a way that is easy for the body to hold its position automatically without your conscious effort.

The surface you sit on should not be cold or hard. Most yoga practitioners sit on a sheepskin or thin padded exercise mat made of natural material such as wool, cotton, or silk. These sitting surfaces provide comfortable seating, sufficient support for the spine, and electromagnetic insulation from the ground. For meditation you can wrap a shawl or blanket around your back and shoulders to keep the spine warm. For this purpose, natural fabrics that do not generate a lot of static electricity are preferred.

able to sit in Easy Pose, an alternative position is sitt up in a chair (Fig. Intro-2). in a chair, remember to chair wisely. The spine must be as straight as possible during meditation, so pick a chair that gives you firm support. A large overstuffed lounge chair may be uncomfortable for a long meditation.

The back of the chair can give you support if it is straight. It is essential that the feet be equally placed flat on the ground to assure that your lower spine and hips do not get out of balance. Do not let the legs hang loosely.

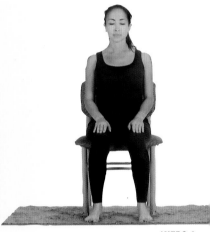

INTRO 2

NECK LOCK

Important: It is a general rule to apply the Neck Lock in all meditations unless otherwise specified.

For proper results in meditation, the spine must be straight from the tailbone to the top of the head. Although you can make most of the spine straight by simply sitting up straight and tall, as described above for Easy Pose, the neck area is not as easy to straighten and thus requires additional attention.

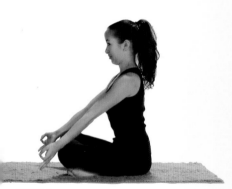

Sit with a straight spine, with one spinal vertebra stacked on top of another, like a stack of coins. The neck vertebrae must also be perfectly straight, and to do that you must take the following action:

With the head facing straight forward, bring the chin directly in towards the Adam's apple as far as possible with a substantial pressure (Fig. Intro-3). This applies a pressure to the back of the neck and aligns the neck vertebrae so they are in line with the rest of the straight spine. The head stays level, tilted neither forward nor backward. This is called Neck Lock, and it regulates the flow of energy and blood into the brain.

INTRO 3

When you practice Kundalini Yoga exercises, energy is generated that can open nerve pathways, which may be blocked, throughout the body. When this blocking happens and is released, there can sometimes be a quick shift in blood pressure causing dizziness. If the Neck Lock is not applied during certain yogic breathing exercises, it can cause uncomfortable pressure in the eyes, ears and heart. Applying Neck Lock regulates these phenomena.

Neck Lock is critically important because it regulates the great flow of energy that is generated in the spine during the practice of Kundalini Yoga, and the energy must flow straight up the spine into the glandular centers of the brain including hypothalamus, pituitary gland and pineal gland. Neck Lock also applies pressure to the parathyroid and thyroid glands, causing them to secrete optimally and stimulate the pituitary, the master endocrine gland. Since the thyroid gland is the guardian of health and youth in the body, Neck Lock has a beneficial healing effect on the body.

DIAPHRAGM LOCK

Diaphragm Lock is applied by lifting the diaphragm up high into the thorax and pulling the upper abdominal muscles back toward the spine (Fig. Intro-4).

This creates a cavity that gives a gentle massage to the intestines and the heart muscles. It is considered to be a powerful lock since it allows the pranic force to transform through the central nerve channel of the

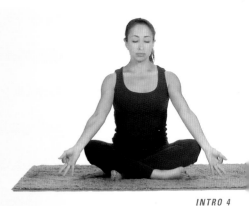

INTRO 4

spine up into the neck region. It also has a direct link to stimulating the hypothalamic-pituitary-adrenal axis in the brain. It stimulates the sense of compassion and can give a new youthfulness to the entire body. The spine should be straight.

Diaphragm Lock is normally applied on the exhale. If applied forcefully on the inhale, it can create uncomfortable pressure in the eyes and heart.

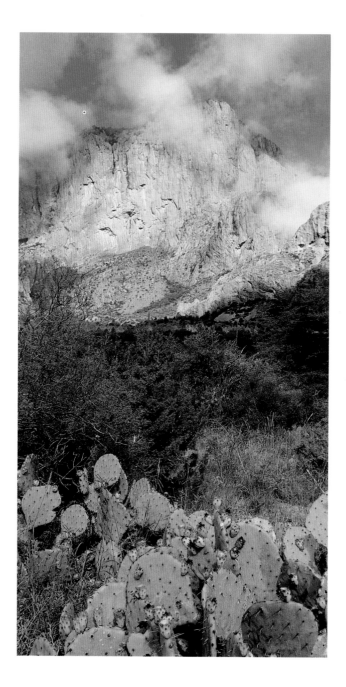

ROOT LOCK OR MOOL BHAND

The Root Lock (also known as mool bhand*) is the most complex of the locks and it is frequently applied. It coordinates and combines the energy of the rectum, sex organs, and navel point.* Mool *is the root, base, or source.*

The first part of the Root Lock is to contract the anal sphincter and draw it in and up as if trying to hold back a bowel movement. Then draw up the sex organ so the urethral tract is contracted. Lastly, pull in the navel point by drawing back the lower abdomen towards the spine so the rectum and sex organs are drawn up toward the navel point (Fig. Intro-4).

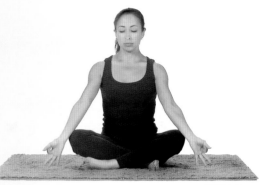

INTRO 4

This action unites the two major energy flows of the body: prana *and* apana. *Prana is the positive, generative energy of the upper body and heart center. Apana is the downward flow of eliminating energy. The Root Lock pulls the apana up and the prana down to the navel point. The combination of the energies generates the psychic heat that can release the Kundalini energy.*

The Root Lock, when applied, is usually applied on the exhale. It sometimes is also applied on the inhale, but only when specified.

GUIDELINES ON PACING YOURSELF

In yoga, each person progresses at their own pace, and gradually develops the physical flexibility to perform the exercises more perfectly. Every yoga exercise is conducted in a controlled and conscious way. It should not physically hurt to do yoga. Most yoga exercise sets take 20 to 30 minutes to complete. Most yoga meditations take between 3 to 11 minutes to complete.

Please be advised that yoga is a discipline that, like martial arts practice forms, should not be altered. There are no exercises in Kundalini Yoga that practitioners invent; all of the technology has been initially taught by Yogi Bhajan and should be practiced exactly as he has taught it. Therefore, if you practice any of the exercises contained herein, you should carefully adhere to the instructions given, including how to Tune In (given below), and you should observe the time duration and/or frequency of practice restrictions stated within the description of each exercise, so that you do not overexert yourself.

For beginners in yoga to develop flexibility and gradually build the capacity to perform the physical exercise sets for the recommended length of time, a good approach is to practice each exercise for only 1 minute (unless less time is specified for that particular exercise), followed by 1 to 3 minutes of relaxation on your back, before doing the next exercise in the set. As you become stronger and better able to perform each exercise, you can, over a period of weeks, extend the duration of each exercise until you achieve the maximum time for each exercise as stated in the instructions in this book. Generally, the first time you practice an exercise set, it will be more difficult than in succeeding sessions. So enjoy the results and don't push yourself; let the body adjust, heal, and grow stronger gradually.

Similarly, for beginners in meditation, start by practicing the meditations in this book for the minimum recommended time, and gradually extend your meditation practice time over a period of weeks or months. If you can make it a habit to practice a particular meditation at a set time of day consistently, results should be more noticeable. You should always consult your physician before beginning this or any other exercise program.

According to ancient yogic tradition, each particular meditation or set of exercises (called a *kriya*), is designed to achieve a particular effect, described in this book under the Benefits section of each such exercise. There is no guarantee that you will achieve the same results. For best results, regular daily practice of yoga is recommended.

Over the last thirty years, modern medical science has begun the process of validating the healing effects of yoga. More than five hundred scientific medical studies have so far been conducted analyzing the effects of yoga and meditation upon a wide range of medical and psychiatric conditions. The results demonstrate that yoga and meditation can have significant positive outcomes in the healing process in almost every medical and psychiatric condition studied to date. The results are encouraging, but much work remains to be done.

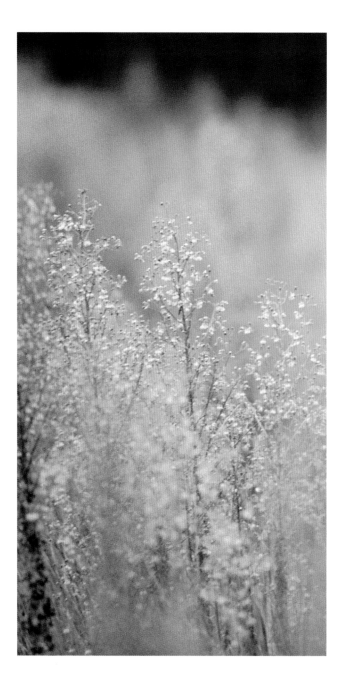

SPECIAL CONSIDERATIONS
FOR WOMEN

During the heaviest menses, avoid strenuous yoga exercises. In particular, do not perform the following exercises either as a solitary exercise or as part of a kriya: Bow Pose, Camel Pose, Locust Pose, Shoulder Stand, Plough Pose, Root Lock, Breath of Fire, strenuous leg lifts, or any pumping of the navel.

Recommendations during pregnancy: In the first three months of pregnancy, you can safely perform regular Kundalini Yoga exercises unless you are not feeling well. After the third month of pregnancy, do not perform Breath of Fire, Diaphragm Lock, Shoulder Stand, Stretch Pose, or any exercises lying on the stomach or that put pressure on the abdomen. Do not perform double leg lifts, although single leg lifts (one leg at a time) may be performed.

Yogi Bhajan has given many recommendations of things to do during pregnancy. For example, Root Lock is good to do. Walk a lot, up to five miles, every day. Several 3HO Foundation books and tapes have been produced on the subject; see the Resources section of this book for contact information.

TUNING IN

The first step in any practice of yoga, or whenever the teachings are shared with anyone, is to tune in to the wisdom within you for guidance and direction.

In the same way that an electrician does not work on electrical wiring with his bare hands, but first puts on insulated gloves and boots, so adequate protection is required when you begin to work with the energy that flows through you.

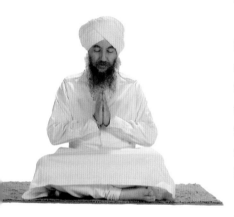

Tuning in links you to the Golden Chain that connects you to your teacher, and from your teacher to his/her teacher, and so on unto Infinity. Even when a trained yoga teacher is present to instruct you, both teacher and student should tune in this way together. Here is how you should tune in:

Sit with a straight spine, eyes closed, hands with palms together in a prayer position in front of the chest. Hands are pressed against the center of the chest, stilling the mind. Inhale deep through the nose and use the full breath to chant aloud:

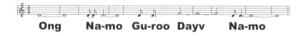

Ong   Na-mo   Gu-roo Dayv   Na-mo

This is pronounced "ohng" (rhymes with sarong), "nam-oh" (rhymes with "ramone"), "goo-roo" (as in "spoon"), "dayv" (rhymes with wave), "nam-oh." This means "I bow to the creative wisdom within, present everywhere, I bow." Loosely translated, it means that you surrender your ego to the creative wisdom within you.

Then inhale deeply and repeat this chant. Then inhale deeply once more and repeat this chant.

Always chant this mantra (quietly and unobtrusively if necessary) three times before practicing any of the yoga and meditation techniques in this book.

Now you can begin to practice yoga.

At the conclusion of your yoga practice, it is customary to sing this song:

May the long time sun shine upon you, all love surround you,

and the pure light within you, guide your way on.

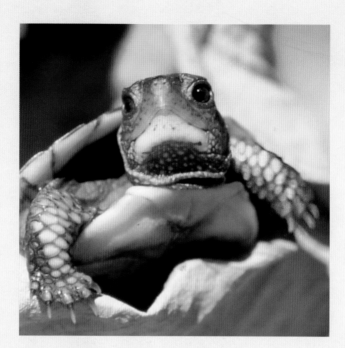

Survival

CHAPTER ONE

Breath to the Rescue

This chapter addresses basic survival skills and shows you how to take control of your life. Applying these techniques can help you to be calm when going into an important interview, or to boost your energy to complete a rush project under a tight deadline.

If you are reading this, you are alive. If you are alive, you are breathing. When you stop breathing, you are no longer alive, and then the things of this life will have no power over you.

So while you are alive, you can relax yourself—or energize yourself—whenever you want, simply by changing your breath pattern. By changing your breathing pattern, you can change your state of mind. This is one of the most basic techniques that yogis use to control and improve their lives. You can do it, too; it is very simple.

A person has one of two problems in life: either they don't have enough energy to do what they want, or they have too much energy and don't know what to do with it. Five minutes of Long Deep Breathing through one or other nostril is all you need to do to change your energy at will.

 Unless otherwise noted, Long Deep Breathing is always done through the nose, not the mouth.

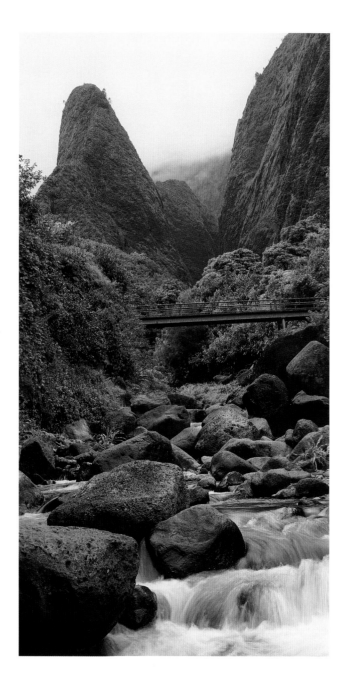

Sit with a straight spine and check your breathing right now. Which nostril are you breathing out of right now? Usually one nostril is clogged up so that you are mainly breathing out of one nostril. Two and a half hours from now, if you check again, you will find that your body has switched nostrils. The body does this automatically to keep your metabolism balanced.

Left nostril breathing lowers the body temperature and lowers the blood pressure. Right nostril breathing raises the body temperature and raises the blood pressure. By cycling the breathing from one nostril to the other every two and a half hours, the body keeps the metabolism cycling like a thermostat. But this cycle does not necessarily match the ordinary eight-hour workday, your eating schedule, the demands of your family, or your social calendar. Sometimes you need an energy level different than the one you may be experiencing at the time.

EXERCISE 1A ❖ TO RELAX

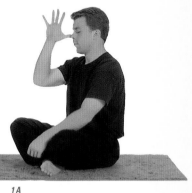

1A

If you are nervous, upset, uptight or stressed out and you want to relax, sit up straight, close off the right nostril, and take twenty-six long deep breaths through the left nostril. On the inhale, fill the stomach with air first, then the lungs from bottom to top. As Figure 1A shows, use the thumb to close off the right nostril while you practice this breathing. Once the lungs are full, pull the navel in toward the spine to push the air out on the exhale.

Use the mantra "Sat Naam" (meaning "truth is my identity," or more simply, "Truth") with the breath: Mentally create the sound "Sat" (rhymes with "but") on the inhale and mentally create the sound "Naam" (rhymes with "mom") on the exhale. After twenty-six long deep breaths, relax. This breathing exercise will take approximately 5 minutes to complete. Now sit quietly and experience how you feel. Then go about your business.

Think of the different situations where you can use this technique. Suppose you are about to go into a very important interview and you are too nervous. Twenty-six long deep breaths through the left nostril is all you need to change your energy, and you can go into that interview relaxed and calm. You can do this quite unobtrusively by pressing your index finger against the outside of your right nostril for twenty-six breaths, and within 5 minutes you will be much more relaxed.

One other simple technique for relieving emotional distress is to drink a glass of water. This changes the water balance in your blood stream, which affects your emotions, and in a little while you'll need to urinate, which is also relaxing. Drinking water is a good way to change your energy after any emotionally stressful situation, including arguments, and it often relieves a headache.

BENEFITS

Relax at will within 5 minutes.

Total Time: 5 minutes

EXERCISE 1B ❖ TO ENERGIZE

If you have low energy, or you are feeling sluggish or depressed, do the same breathing exercise as above but close off the left nostril and take twenty-six long deep breaths through the right nostril (instead of the left nostril). This will raise your energy level and stimulate your physical energy, charge you up with vitality, wake you up, and give you the energy you need to go about your business.

Suppose you have some important work to accomplish under a tight deadline, but you are feeling tired, worn out, and uninspired. Twenty-six long deep breaths through the right nostril (Fig. 1B) will charge you up with physical vitality, and you will have the energy and momentum to get the work done.

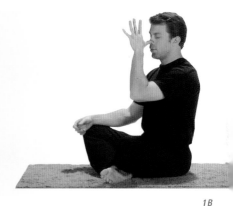

1B

BENEFITS
Energize whenever you need to, within 5 minutes.
Total Time: 5 minutes

Long Deep Breathing can change your destiny, because it puts your energy under your conscious control.

Expanding Lung Capacity

The normal person breathes about fifteen or sixteen breaths per minute. If you can expand your lung capacity through regular practice of yogic Long Deep Breathing techniques, such as the Basic Breath Series (Exercise 1C) shown here, you can gradually lower the average number of breaths per minutes required to oxygenate your blood. By slowing down the rate of breath, you will calm the mind.

Yogis know that the state of mind is directly affected by the rate of breath. Slow the breath rate, and you force the mind to become more calm. When you are calm and centered, no matter how hectic the circumstances around you, you will be more effective in thinking and in action.

The lung capacity of an average adult is about 6,000 cubic centimeters, but typically only 600–700 cubic centimeters capacity is used for normal breathing. Through practice of yogic Long Deep Breathing, this normal breathing capacity can be significantly increased. Most people breathe shallowly, using only the top one-third of their full lung capacity. If you do not expand the lungs to their full capacity the small air sacks (alveoli) in the lungs cannot clean their mucous lining properly. Therefore, if you do not get enough oxygen, you gradually accumulate toxic irritants and environmental pollutants in the lungs that lead to infections and disease buildup. However, if you develop the habit of breathing deeply throughout the day, you will clean the lungs and will take, on average, fewer breaths per minute.

According to the yogis, if you can lower the breath rate to eight breaths per minute, then you gain self-control. You will be able to control your action and reaction to external events and internal feelings.

If you can lower the breath rate to four breaths per minute, then you can know the past, present and future. Your intuition will compute for you exactly the right action to take in any circumstance, and you can know in advance the outcome of any sequence of action you may start. Thus your actions come into harmony with the universe.

Gradually expand your lung capacity, your tolerance and endurance by regular practice of the Basic Breath Series. Long chanting of "Sat Naam" at the conclusion of this exercise, or by itself, opens you up to new experience. If you are feeling lost or hopeless, chanting "Sat Naam" is a good way to heal.

EXERCISE 1C ❖ BASIC BREATH SERIES

This series introduces you to your breath, the source of life. The yogic name for breathing exercises is pranayam. *The* prana, *the life force that comes to you in the breath, is the life force of the atom. It is not a small thing. Through control of the breath, you gain control of your mind.*

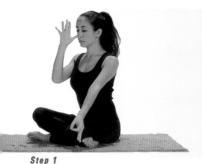

Sit in Easy Pose with a straight spine. Make an antenna of the right-hand fingers and block the right nostril with the thumb. Begin Long Deep Breathing through the left nostril for 3 minutes. Inhale and hold the breath for 10 seconds.

Step 1

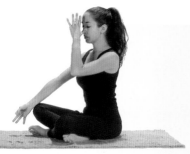

Repeat the first step, but use the left hand and breathe through the right nostril. Continue for 3 minutes. Inhale and hold the breath for 10 seconds.

Step 2

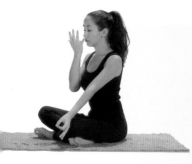

Inhale through the left nostril, exhale through the right using long deep breaths. Use the thumb and little finger of the right hand to close alternate nostrils. Continue for 3 minutes.

Step 3

Repeat Step 3 except inhale through the right nostril and exhale through the left. Use the thumb and little finger of the left hand to close alternate nostrils. Continue for 3 minutes.

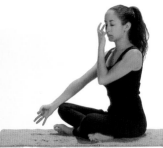

Step 4

Sit in Easy Pose with hands in Gyan Mudra (on each hand, touch the tips of the index finger and thumb together). Begin Breath of Fire (see Exercise 1D for instructions). Totally center yourself at the brow point (on the forehead slightly above where the root of the nose meets the eyebrows). Continue with a regular powerful breath for up to 7½ minutes. Then inhale, circulating the energy. Then relax or meditate for 5 minutes.

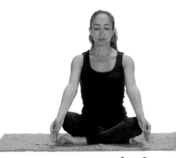

Step 5

Sit up straight and chant aloud a prolonged "Sat Naam" once on each breath for a few minutes. This sound opens you up to new experience.

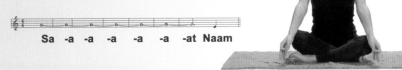

Sa -a -a -a   -a   -a -at Naam

Step 6

BENEFITS

This set opens the pranic channels and balances the breath in the two sides of your body. It is often practiced before a more strenuous physical kriya. It is great to do by itself whenever you need a quick lift and a clear mind.

Total Time: 23 minutes

EXERCISE 1D ❖ BREATH OF FIRE

One of the most effective breathing exercises for healing the body is the Breath of Fire.

Breath of Fire is used consistently throughout the Kundalini Yoga kriyas. It is very important that Breath of Fire be practiced and mastered by the yoga practitioner.

Sit in Easy Pose, a comfortable cross-legged position with a straight spine, with the hands in Gyan Mudra and the eyes closed.

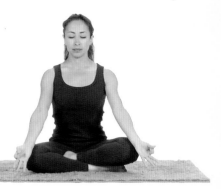

1D

In Breath of Fire, the focus of energy is at the navel point. The breath is through the nose and fairly rapid (two to three breaths per second), continuous and powerful with no pause between the inhale and exhale. As you exhale, the air is pushed out by pulling the navel point and abdomen in towards the spine. In this motion, the chest area is moderately relaxed. As you inhale, use the forward thrust of the navel point to bring the air into the lungs. This is a very balanced breath with no emphasis on either the exhale or inhale, and with equal power given to both.

Check to make sure Breath of Fire is done correctly by placing your hand on the navel point to feel it moving in and out.

BENEFITS

Breath of Fire is a cleansing breath that cleans the blood and releases old toxins from the lungs, mucous lining, blood vessels, and cells. Breath of Fire strengthens the nervous system and stimulates the glandular system. Regular practice expands the lung capacity. You can start practicing with 3 minutes of Breath of Fire at a sitting and over a period of weeks gradually build your capacity to practice Breath of Fire for 20 minutes continuously. Begin by alternating 3 minutes of Breath of Fire with 2 minutes of rest for five complete sets of breath and relaxation.

Total Time: 3–25 minutes

EXERCISE 1E ✤ COOLING BREATH

This Cooling Breath, known as Sitali Kriya, *is a healing breath useful in ridding the body of illness.*

Sit in Easy Pose with a straight spine (Fig. 1E1). Take the tongue and roll it into a **V**, with the tip just outside of the lips (Fig. 1E2). Inhale deeply through the rolled tongue, exhale through the nose. Continue for a minimum of 2 to 3 minutes.

1E1

1E2

BENEFITS

This kriya gives you power, strength, and vitality. It detoxifies the body and relieves anger. It is helpful to practice it whenever you get a fever, sickness, or discomfort. According to ancient yogic tradition, it is a cure within you. At first the tongue will be bitter, then it will become sweet. Once it becomes sweet, you will have overcome all sickness inside. Sitali Kriya is good to do for twenty-six breaths in the morning and twenty-six breaths in the evening.

Total Time: At least 2 minutes

People who practice this kriya are said to have all things come to them that they need by the planetary ether. In mystical terms, you are served by the heavens.

EXERCISE 1F ❖ ASTHMA RELIEF

Asthma has become a much more common ailment in the world due to the proliferation of pollutants in the air and environment. If you have this problem, try the Asthma Relief exercise.

Stand up. Put the heels together. Extend the hands overhead, arms straight up, palms together. Lean back as far as possible. Do Breath of Fire for 1 to 3 minutes. To prevent injury, have a soft bed behind you in case you lose your balance. To end this exercise, inhale and stand up straight, and relax the breath, relaxing the arms by your sides.

1F

BENEFITS
Although there is no hand clapping in this exercise, Yogi Bhajan says asthma "runs away like a crow at the clap of your hands" with this exercise.
Total Time: 1–3 minutes

CHAPTER TWO
Deeply Relaxed

We all want to be free of stress, but few people know how to achieve it.

In the early days of microcomputing and during the second year that I worked at the company, we opened one of the world's first business-to-business retail computer stores in central Phoenix, Arizona. My job was sales, but I didn't know anything about how to sell professionally. I was enthusiastic about the technology and could get potential customers who walked in the door interested in what these little computers could do. But it was months before we got any formal sales training, and it was a stressful time for me. John, on the other hand, knew what to do.

John Lebesque was our best salesperson. He had several years experience in selling minicomputers and he was a polished professional salesperson. The thing that amazed me was how calm he seemed. He was low-key and friendly, in contrast to my high-pitched intensity. I could not figure out how he managed to deal with all the stress and uncertainty associated with selling, and I admired his calmness in the face of it.

Then one day John did not show up for work. He was in the hospital with a bad ulcer, and he never came back to our company. Meanwhile, I was doing yoga every morning before coming to work to deal with my stress. John just suppressed his stress, and it ruined his health.

I wish I had known then about this quick but very effective meditation (Meditation 2A)—I would have recommended it for John. It is so easy to do, and gives quick relief.

MEDITATION 2A ❖ MEDITATION TO QUELL AN AGITATED MIND

Sit in Easy Pose with a straight spine. If you are sitting on a chair, make sure your feet are flat on the ground, and the legs are not crossed.

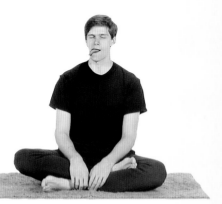

Open the mouth to make an **O**. Stick the tongue out of the right side of the mouth, to form a **Q**. Keep the tongue out. If you have trouble holding the tongue in this position, hold it slightly between the teeth. (Note: The tongue should *not* be straight out, but extended out to the right side of the mouth.) Your **Q** should be perfect.

Breathe long and deeply through the mouth, keeping the tongue extended the whole time. The eyes are closed. You can play any beautiful music.

To end the exercise: Holding the position, inhale and hold the breath for 13 seconds, then squeeze the breath out with a powerful exhale through the sides of the mouth. Then repeat by inhaling and holding the breath for 11 seconds and then exhale out, and then one last time, inhale and hold 7 seconds and exhale out. Relax.

2A

BENEFITS

You must watch how to avoid death and be extra healthy. There is no more powerful relaxation than this. When you are very nervous, and you have so many thoughts, and you are being ground up by everything, do this for 3 minutes. You will be shocked—things will disappear. There's nothing more relaxing. —*Yogi Bhajan*

Total Time: 3 minutes

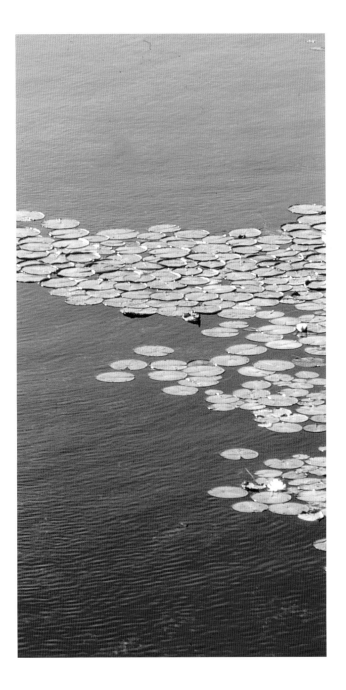

EXERCISE 2B ✣ GUIDED RELAXATION

Another effective technique for developing a relaxed state of mind is the guided relaxation. This technique is often used in regular yoga classes following completion of strenuous exercises. However, it is useful anytime you have about 30 minutes to relax and doze off. It is very healing.

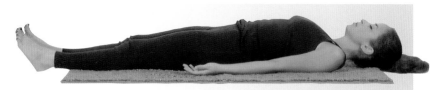

2B

Lie down on the back comfortably (Fig. 2B), with the arms by the sides, palms facing up. Pick up one foot and drop it; wherever it falls, let it lie there and don't move it. Pick up the other foot and drop it. Lift up one arm and drop it by your side. Lift up the other arm and drop it by your side. Lift the head up an inch and drop it. Focus the attention at the brow point, slightly above where the root of the nose meets the eyebrows. When the body inhales, mentally create the sound "Sat," meaning truth, and, when the body exhales, mentally create the sound "Naam," meaning identity. Truth is my identity.

Now feel the feet. Feel how they feel. Feel all the energy that's there. Now relax the feet, and draw all the energy up to the brow point, mentally inhaling "Sat" and exhaling "Naam" with every breath.

Feel the ankles and the lower legs up to the knees. Feel how they feel. Feel all the energy that's there. Now relax the lower legs, and draw all the energy up to the brow point, mentally inhaling "Sat" and exhaling "Naam" with every breath.

Feel the legs from the knees up to the hips. Feel how they feel. Feel all the energy that's there. Now relax the upper legs, and draw all the energy up to the brow point, mentally inhaling "Sat" and exhaling "Naam" with every breath.

Feel the torso from the hips and buttocks, the sex organ, the internal organs, the back, the ribs, the lungs and heart. Feel how they feel. Feel all the energy that's there. Now relax the torso from the hips and buttocks, and the internal organs, and the back, all the way up to the rib cage, the lungs and heart, and draw all the energy up to the brow point, mentally inhaling "Sat" and exhaling "Naam" with every breath.

Feel the fingers and hands. Feel how they feel. Feel all the energy that's there. Now relax the hands, and draw all the energy up to the brow point, mentally inhaling "Sat" and exhaling "Naam" with every breath.

Feel the forearms from the wrists up to the elbows. Feel how they feel. Feel all the energy that's there. Now relax the forearms, and draw all the energy up to the brow point, mentally inhaling "Sat" and exhaling "Naam" with every breath.

Feel the upper arms up to the shoulders. Feel how they feel. Feel all the energy that's there. Now relax the upper arms and shoulders, and draw all the energy up to the brow point, mentally inhaling "Sat" and exhaling "Naam" with every breath.

Feel the neck and jaw, the teeth and tongue, the cheeks and eyes and eyebrows and forehead, the back of the head, the ears and hair. Feel how they feel. Feel all the energy that's there. Now relax the neck and jaw and face and eyes and forehead and ears and hair, and draw all the energy up to the brow point, mentally inhaling "Sat" and exhaling "Naam" with every breath.

Imagine sitting on the bank of a river, watching it flow by. The river of life, and everything that is happening, is just flowing by. Begin throwing the sounds into the river, "Sat" on the inhale and "Naam" on the exhale with every breath. Just sink into the earth, relax, and watch the breath, "Sat" on the inhale and "Naam" on the exhale with every breath.

After mentally guiding yourself through this relaxation, you may fall asleep. If so, you can wake up after about 15 to 30 minutes of relaxation.

BENEFITS
Complete relaxation for the entire body.
Total Time: 15-30 minutes

MEDITATION 2C ❖ PITTAR KRIYA, MEDITATION TO ELIMINATE STRESS

Sit in Easy Pose with a straight spine.

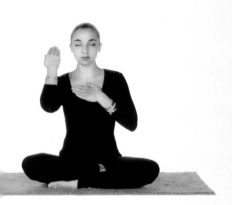

Put the left palm at center of the chest (on the heart center); right elbow bent, the right hand, cupped, moves past the right ear, as if throwing water back behind you over the shoulder.

Keep the right arm moving back and forth, making sure that the wrist passes the right ear, for 11 minutes.

No particular breathing pattern is specified, so breathe through the nose as necessary. Time is to be exact. Not less, not more. Then inhale deeply, hold the breath while pressing the right arm as far back behind as possible. Repeat the inhale and hold twice more. Relax.

2C

BENEFITS

This kriya eliminates stress and cleans the liver. This kriya works on stress. Do this meditation if you want to feel relaxed, mellow, and able to handle the pressures of each day.

Total Time: Exactly 11 minutes

CHAPTER THREE

Sleep

One day I was having lunch with Jamal Malamud, one of our computer store franchise owners from California, during our annual convention. The convention was always the highlight of the business year for me because it was a chance to meet old friends and catch up.

It had been a year of tremendous growth for Jamal, with more staff, expanded product and service offerings, and more large corporate clients than ever. Although things were going well, Jamal could no longer sleep at night. The pressures of his expanded business were enormous, and he was lying awake every night worrying about things. So for months, he had been sleeping fitfully or not at all. This was taking a big toll on his health, and he was often irritable with people from lack of sleep.

I shared with Jamal this simple exercise (Exercise 3A) for falling asleep quickly and suggested he try it.

A year later, we met again at the next annual convention. "I sleep every night, and everything is going great," he told me. "This one exercise changed my whole life. I thank you, and my whole family thanks you."

After that, whenever I discovered a business associate was having trouble sleeping due to worries, I just told them about Jamal's results. I would say, "Don't take my word for it—just ask Jamal!"

EXERCISE 3A ❖ HOW TO FALL ASLEEP

Sometimes you lie awake and the mind races with thoughts and worries, and you can't fall asleep. Try this exercise for a few minutes, and you should be able to drop right off to sleep.

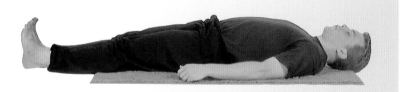

3A1

Lying on your back and keeping your heels on the bed, breathe long and deeply through the nose. On the inhale, stretch the toes toward your head while mentally chanting "Sat" (Fig. 3A1).

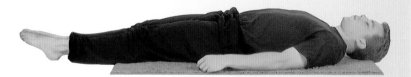

3A2

On the exhale, stretch the toes toward the bed away from your head while mentally chanting "Naam" (Fig. 3A2). Continue for 3 to 5 minutes, then just relax and go to sleep.

BENEFITS

Fall asleep whenever you need to.
Total Time: 3–5 minutes

EXERCISE 3B ❖ SLEEP SUBSTITUTE

Sometimes you don't have time to sleep, but need to catch some rest quickly. Some of the world's greatest leaders had the ability to rejuvenate themselves by taking short naps whenever they needed some sleep, George Washington and Napoleon among them. For those of us who don't have that ability, Shoulder Stand is the next best thing.

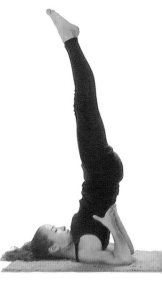

Lie on the back, bring the spine and legs straight up to as nearly a vertical position as possible, and support the buttocks with the arms. Your weight is supported by the elbows and shoulders. Relax in this position and breathe long and deeply through the nose.

3B

BENEFITS

15 minutes of Shoulder Stand is equivalent to 2 hours of sleep for the relaxation it gives you. Shoulder Stand is not a replacement for regular sleep, but can be a good substitute when your schedule does not allow for the sleep you need. Suggested time: 15–30 minutes, for the equivalent of up to 4 hours of sleep relaxation.

Total Time: 15–30 minutes

MEDITATION 3C ❖ RESTFUL REFRESHING SLEEP

You can do the following meditation, Shabd Kriya, before going to bed to help you enter into a deep, restful sleep so you can wake up refreshed.

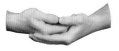

Sit in any comfortable posture with the spine straight. Place the hands in the lap, palms up with the right hand over the left. The thumbs are together and point forward (Fig. 3C1).

3C1

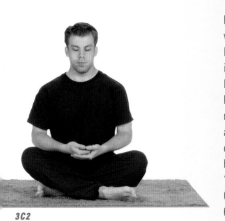

Focus the eyes on the tip of the nose, with the eyelids half-closed (Fig. 3C2). Inhale in four equal parts, mentally reciting one syllable of the mantra "Saa Taa Naa Maa" on each part of the inhale. Hold the breath, mentally reciting the mantra "Saa Taa Naa Maa" four times for a total of sixteen beats. Exhale in two equal strokes, mentally reciting "Wah-hay" on the first exhale stroke and "Guroo" on the second exhale stroke. Continue this breathing pattern for 15 to 62 minutes.

3C2

"Saa Taa Naa Maa" is the mantra "Sat Naam" (meaning "Truth") broken down into its component sounds. This mantra cleanses the subconscious mind. "Wah-hay Guroo" means "Infinite Wisdom."
The best time to practice this kriya is every night before bed.

BENEFITS

If it is practiced regularly, sleep will be deep and relaxed and the nerves will regenerate. After a few months, the rhythm of your breath as you sleep will be subconsciously regulated in the same rhythm! You will think better, work better, share better, love better, and exercise better. This rhythmic mantra will eventually progress so that even in daily activities you will automatically hear the mantra and take on the breath rhythm. This confirms the vibratory effect of the meditation within you and suffuses its healing energy into your surroundings.

Total Time: 15–62 minutes

 There cannot be enough praise of this meditation and its growth promoting effect on the personality. It gives you personal radiance and the radiance gives patience, which is the first condition of real love. Being patient, you can work with others without attention to their mistakes, as the sun gives light and warmth to all people. The incorporation of this practical warmth and universality in the personality comes with the disciplined practice of Shabd Kriya.

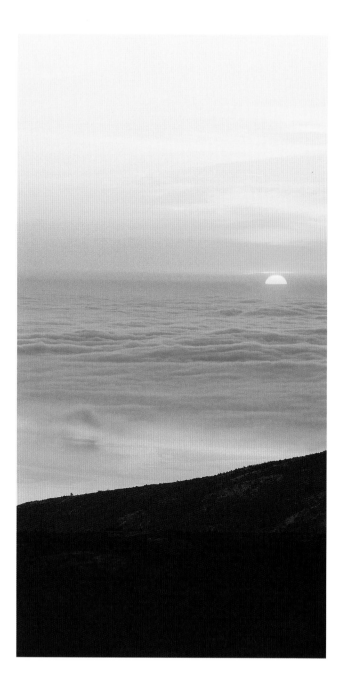

The Yogi Way to Get Up in the Morning

One of the best ways to combat sickness is a daily cold shower. This form of hydrotherapy improves your circulation, cleanses the bloodstream and rejuvenates all the internal organs. The process is described in detail in Step 8 of the recommended daily wakeup practice (Exercise 3D). For overall optimum health and well being, this is the yogi way to get up in the morning.

A cold shower in the morning has been my regular practice for nearly thirty years; I think it is one of the main reasons I rarely ever get sick.

EXERCISE 3D HOW TO GET UP IN THE MORNING

"When you wake, tell yourself you are bountiful, blissful, and beautiful."

—Yogi Bhajan

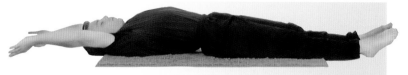

Step 1

1. SPINE STRETCH

Always come out of sleep slowly and gradually, so that you don't create a shock to your nervous system. Lying down and keeping the eyes closed, inhale deeply with the arms up and over the head. Take a few long deep breaths through the nose, stretching the spine on each breath.

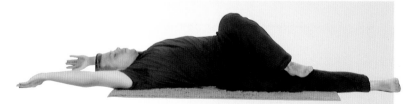

Step 2

2. CAT STRETCH

With both arms still above the head and on the bed, keep the eyes closed and bend one knee up to the chest and swing it across the front of the body to touch the bed on the opposite side, tucking the foot behind the knee of the leg that is straight, and keeping both shoulders on the bed. Arch and stretch the back like a cat does before it gets up. Twist and turn and bend to the maximum. Then do the same stretch on the other side of the body with the other knee. This is good for your circulation and for the nervous system; it balances the body's electromagnetic field and enables you to go through the day balanced and calm.

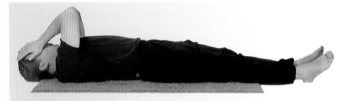

Step 3

3. PALM THE EYES

Now, lying flat on the back, put the palms of the hands tightly over your closed eyes. Then open the eyes and look directly into the palms of the hands. Slowly continue to gaze at the palms as you lift the hands straight up to about eighteen inches above the face. This gives the optic nerve a chance to adjust gradually to the light, and helps to keep your eyesight strong. To protect your eyesight, avoid any sudden shock of light as you get up in the morning.

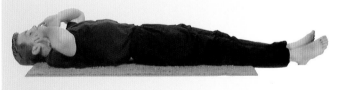

Step 4

4. FACE MASSAGE

From the eighteen-inch height, bring the fingertips down to the center of the forehead, and with a circular motion, massage the forehead from the center out to the temples and down both sides of the face to the tip of the chin. Then massage the nose and the ears, squeeze the nostrils and the earlobes briefly to get the circulation going. Take a few more long deep breaths through the nose to open up the lungs.

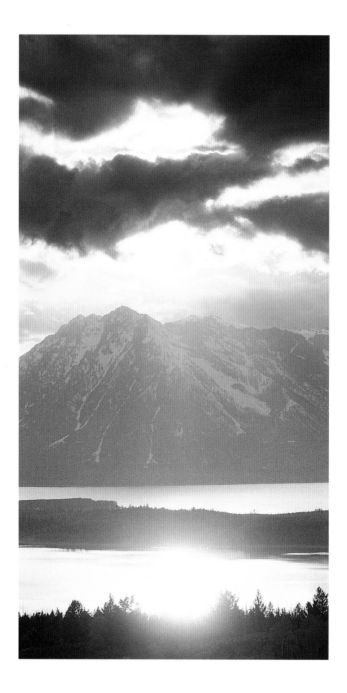

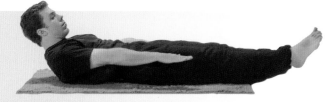

Step 5

5. STRETCH POSE

Lie on the back and come up into Stretch Pose: head and feet up six inches off the ground, balanced at the navel point, arms up six inches and straight with fingers pointed toward the toes and palms down, and stare at the toes. Breath of Fire for 1 minute. Mentally inhale "Sat" and exhale "Naam" with every breath. This exercise adjusts the entire nervous system as all 72,000 major nerves flow through the navel point and are coordinated there. It also moves the pulse directly under the navel to center the physical body. Relax on your back for 15 seconds (don't fall back to sleep!) and prepare for the next exercise.

6. NOSE TO KNEES

Bend both knees to the chest, hold them tight against the body, lift the head and put the nose right in between the knees. In this position do Breath of Fire for 30 seconds to 1 minute, pumping the navel. This stimulates the apana (outgoing life breath) and helps your elimination system. The Breath of Fire purifies the blood and gets rid of tox-

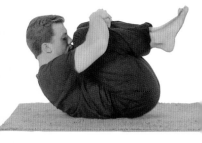

Step 6

ins. Then inhale deeply, exhale, and relax the breath as you do the next exercise.

7. RELAX THE HEART

Keeping the knees tightly clasped to the chest, turn briefly onto the right side and rest for a minute or two. This posture strengthens the heart. Don't fall asleep because there is more to do.

According to Yogi Bhajan, to stay awake during your morning yogic exercises, a cold shower is the best way to start the day and strengthen your nervous system, glandular system, and circulatory system. Another great benefit of a daily cold shower is that you will almost never get sick.

8. HYDROTHERAPY

Men should wear some kind of support for the gonads while taking a shower. Women should wear shorts or underwear that covers the thighs. Before getting in the shower, massage your body all over with a little almond oil. When the cold water hits the surface of the skin, blood from deep inside the body rushes to the surface, improving your circulation. This is called hydrotherapy and it strengthens your entire nervous system. Vigorously rub your body with your hands to stimulate the circulation.

Go in and out of the water four times, constantly massaging your body until the water no longer feels cold. Be sure to get the armpits (major nerve centers) and the insides of the thighs. Women should massage the breasts during the cold shower.

Turn off the water and dry off briskly with a rough towel to further stimulate your circulation. Then put on loose comfortable exercise clothing, and you are ready to do your morning *sadhana*, your personal daily spiritual practice.

BENEFITS

Maximize your health on a daily basis by starting your day the yogi way.

Total Time: 7 minutes for Steps 1–7

CHAPTER FOUR

Headache Relief

Angela Fantazzi was a sprightly twenty-year-old daughter of Perry Fantazzi, one of our franchise owners from New York. We got to talking one night during the annual convention at a party where the live band music was so loud it hurt your ears and made it nearly impossible to have a conversation.

We stepped outside, and as we talked about how painful the loud music was, Angela started telling me about the painful chronic headaches she had been getting several times a month for the past year. Her doctors could find nothing wrong with her and suggested over-the-counter painkillers as a way to cope.

Being otherwise young and healthy, she could not figure out any correlation of headaches to her activity, work, exercise, menstrual cycle, or eating patterns. I am not medically trained so could only offer a yogic suggestion that she try Bridge Pose (Exercise 4) for 3 minutes on a daily basis, and whenever she had a headache. That, plus drink a glass or two of water whenever she felt a headache coming on.

A year later, I met Angela again at the next convention. Her headaches were gone. She had practiced the Bridge Pose exercise for 3 minutes daily and as needed during the year, and eventually her headaches had ceased. She was happy to be living a normal life again.

EXERCISE 4 ❖ HEADACHE RELIEF

When you are weak, or have a headache, do Bridge Pose:

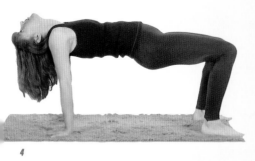

Sit up with legs out straight in front. Brace the arms on the ground behind the waist. Raise the body up so the torso is parallel to the ground. Allow the head to drop back. Long Deep Breathing (ten or twenty breaths) for 3 minutes can relieve any headache. Keep the navel point pressed up. To end, inhale deeply and hold for 12 seconds. Circulate this breath in the body. Then relax.

4

BENEFITS

This exercise helps to relieve headaches.

If you want to fall asleep quickly and soundly, do Bridge Pose for 15 minutes, then relax.

Total Time: 3 minutes

If you suffer from headaches, you might consider allergies as a possible cause. See your physician for testing or contact Great Smokies Diagnostic Laboratory, listed in the Resources section of this book.

CHAPTER FIVE
Stamina to Keep Up

My wife was in labor fifty-one hours giving birth to our son. By the forty-eighth hour, we had both been awake continuously without any sleep, and I was exhausted—but the process was not over. She was exhausted too, but had no trouble staying awake because the contractions were so frequent. I was desperate for some way to reinvigorate, and fortunately recalled having recently practiced the exercise for Rejuvenating the Nervous System (Meditation 5).

In twelve minutes, I was reenergized and ready to continue. Three hours later, he was born, strong and alert, but also quite tired after such a prolonged process.

I recommend this exercise to anyone who needs a big energy boost when it seems impossible to keep going.

MEDITATION 5 ❖ REJUVENATE THE NERVOUS SYSTEM

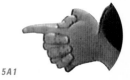

5A1

Sit in Easy Pose with a straight spine. Interlace the three fingers of the hands and put the two Jupiter (index) fingers straight out and the thumbs, the representatives of the ego, crossing over each other (Fig. 5A1).

The idea behind placing your hands in this position is that the meridian of the left and the right sides shall join and be neutralized in all areas of consciousness, except in the area of awareness. The index finger represents awareness, and it relates to the second area of the brain, which gives you an intuitive nature.

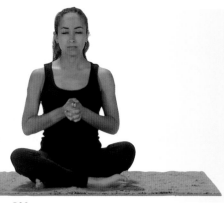

Now close the eyes totally and look exactly 90 degrees straight out to the horizon (Fig. 5A2). It will not take more than 3 minutes to bring you to a stability of mental consciousness. Through closed eyes, look straight ahead, with the joined hands locked in the center near the heart.

5A2

After 3 minutes, begin a 9-minute cycle of creating the sound of

Saa Taa Naa Maa

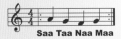

Saa Taa Naa Maa

in a powerful whisper (Figs. 5A3 and 5A4). After 9 minutes, inhale and hold the breath, and concentrate on the spine, from the tailbone to the top. Then let it go, relax, and observe yourself.

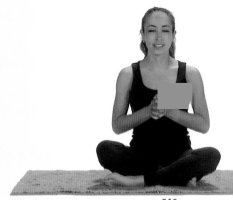

5A3

Nine minutes is the time required to change the entire nervous condition of a person. The most powerful energy in the individual is in the nervous system—and you can shape up the nervous system in 9 minutes! If you honestly maintain the rhythm and the powerful breath with the whisper of "Saa Taa Naa Maa," then you can do it.

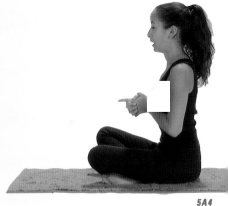

5A4

You may practice this meditation for longer than the minimum 12 minutes. If this is done for 2½ hours, exactly and perfectly, then in a short period of weeks, depending upon one's individual construction, it can put you at the level of a very powerful, intuitive person.

BENEFITS

This exercise will bring you out of depression and nervousness, and will bring you to a neutral state of consciousness. It takes almost 5 minutes for a man to bring his total regenerative energy under his own creative control. By doing this chant, we bring the breath rhythm from fifteen to eight, which is the most effective pranayam ever known in the science of regeneration.

Total Time: 12 minutes

CHAPTER SIX Healing

Yoga is a total healing system. Here is a meditation that invokes the healing power within you.

MEDITATION 6A ❧ HEALING THE PHYSICAL, MENTAL, AND SPIRITUAL BODIES

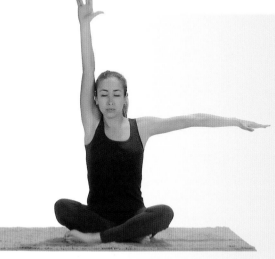

6A1

Sit in Easy Pose with the spine straight, chin in, chest out. Raise the right arm straight up with the palm facing forward. Stretch the left arm out to the side parallel to the floor with the palm facing down. Separate the fingers of each hand so that the Sun (ring) and Mercury (little) fingers are together, and the Jupiter (index) and Saturn (middle) fingers are together (Fig. 6A1). Close the eyes and meditate for 11 minutes maximum.

To finish: Inhale deeply and hold the breath in for 10 seconds, stretching the arms and tightening the entire body. Exhale and repeat this sequence two more times.

Your body will start healing itself after the first 3 minutes. Your entire cellular system will interact to heal you. To practice this meditation, alternate the arm positions each day. The first day, practice with the right arm up and the left arm out to the side; the next day stretch the left arm up and the right arm out to the side (Fig. 6A2); and so on.

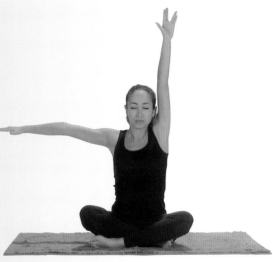

6A2

You must always keep the elbows straight to get the benefits of this exercise. If you would like a mantra to use with this meditation, Yogi Bhajan has recommended the mantra: Har Haray Haree, Wah-hay Guroo.

The "r" sound in this mantra is not pronounced exactly like the normal American "r." While making this "r" sound, the tongue flicks the upper palate in the same way it does making the "t" sound in the word "kitty."

BENEFITS

Body shall start healing and every muscle shall start hurting. This is central nervous system control therapy. In exactly 11 minutes, your entire cellular system shall change. This is the most powerful self-purification you can do. It can give you complete control of your being. It improves intuition and makes you

powerful and healthy. You'll be free of all garbage: physical, mental, and spiritual. After forty days it will start working on your subtle bodies. Whatever starts happening to you after forty days, keep it to yourself. Don't speak of it to anyone.

—*Yogi Bhajan*

Total Time: Up to 11 minutes maximum

EXERCISE 6B ✵ STRONG DIGESTIVE SYSTEM

If your digestive system is strong, you can go through almost any kind of stress and survive. When you are under stress, one thing you should do is reduce the volume of food you consume. This helps to conserve your energy and reduces the possibility of developing digestive problems.

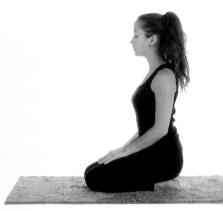

One of the simplest exercises for improving digestion is sitting in Rock Pose (Fig. 6B), also called Vajrasan or Perfect Pose. Just sit up straight on the heels.

6B

BENEFITS

Yogis say that you can digest anything in Rock Pose, even rocks. It can provide relief in cases of minor digestive stress or overeating.

Total Time: 5–31 minutes

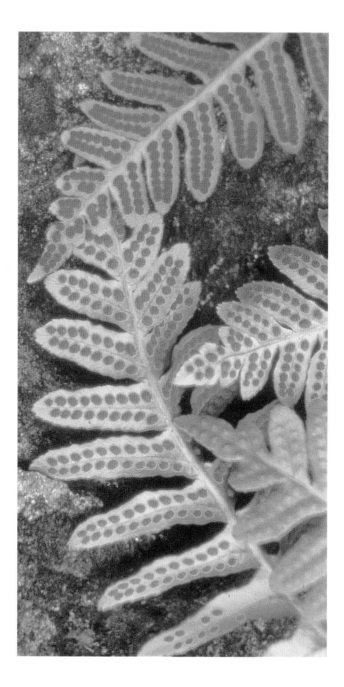

Three Sacred Roots

Garlic, onions, and ginger are the three sacred roots of the yogis. If you include them regularly in your diet, cooked or raw, they will serve to gradually improve your health. One tasty way to combine these ingredients is in a curry that can be eaten with boiled or steamed rice, other sautéed vegetables, and fresh yogurt. See *The Golden Temple Vegetarian Cookbook,* by Yogi Bhajan, for the Trinity Root Curry (basic masala) and other related recipes.

Garlic is an antibacterial medicinal herb that increases your sexual potency, strengthens the glandular system, tonifies the nervous system, and lowers the blood pressure. It is an aid to digestion and eliminates parasites and harmful microorganisms from the digestive tract.

Onion is a blood purifier that helps the body eliminate toxins. It is an aid to digestion.

Ginger tonifies the nervous system, stimulates the cerebral-spinal fluid, stimulates digestion, and stimulates the glandular system.

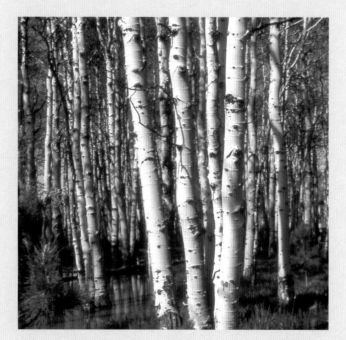

Security

CHAPTER SEVEN
Overcoming Fear and Phobias

I used to be scared of heights. While it is always exciting to see a new skyline from the hotel room in a city not visited before, I did not enjoy getting up close to the window to look straight down. I used to get weak in the knees and feeling dizzy and off-balance while looking down. It always amazed me to see pictures of workers walking along the steel girders of high-rise buildings under construction.

Then I found out about Pranam Mudra (Meditation 7B). Practice this 9-minute exercise forty times within a 24-hour period to resolve child-hood fears and phobias. Pranam Mudra works on the magnetic field to clear many kinds of negative imprints and traumas from your subconscious, such as fear of crowds, claustrophobia, and fear of authority figures. So don't be intimidated by the Boss: do Pranam Mudra.

One year I practiced this exercise forty times on my birthday as a yogic gift to myself. After that, the deep fear reaction that I used to have to heights disappeared. I can't say that I am fond of heights, but at least they no longer make me dizzy with fright.

Here is how I programmed the day: Each exercise takes 9 minutes; with a 6-minute layout on the back, that makes it possible to do the exercise four times per hour. I started in the morning and did 5 hours, then rested an hour for lunch, then completed 5 more hours. Happy Birthday!

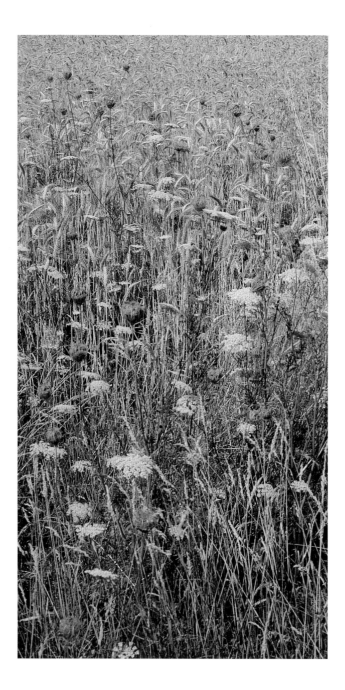

EXERCISE 7A ✤ ARCHER POSE

Archer Pose helps develop your courage, stamina, and nerve strength.

Stand in Archer Pose with the left leg bent forward so the left knee is over the toes. The right leg is straight back with the foot flat on the ground, at a 45-degree angle to the front foot. Raise the left arm straight in front, parallel to the ground, and make a fist as if grasping a bow. Pull the right arm back as if pulling the bowstring back to the right shoulder. Feel a tension across the chest. Face forward and fix the eyes above the fist to the horizon (Fig. 7A1). About 70 percent of the weight is on the forward leg. Hold this position with Long Deep Breathing through the nose for 1 to 3 minutes.

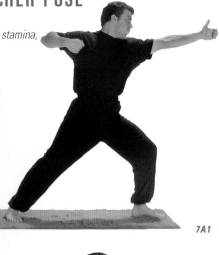

7A1

Then switch sides so the Archer Pose is with the right leg bent forward, and hold this position (Fig. 7A2) for the same duration (1–3 minutes) with Long Deep Breathing through the nose.

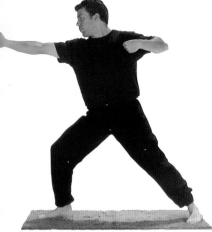

7A2

BENEFITS

Archer Pose applies a pressure to every cell in the body and strengthens the entire nervous system. By applying a stretch to the sex nerve that runs along the inner thighs, this exercise stimulates your potency to develop courage.

Total Time: 2–6 minutes

MEDITATION 7B ❖ PRANAM MUDRA

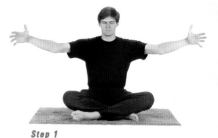

Step 1

1. Sit in Easy Pose with a straight spine with the arms spread wide as if to receive someone in your arms. Use a powerful breath for powerful effect. Tense the fingers, letting all the tension and pressure exist in the fingers, while practicing Long Deep Breathing through the nose for 1 minute. Make the fingers strong as steel.

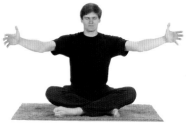

Step 2

2. Over the next 1 minute, continue Long Deep Breathing as you very slowly bring the hands together until they are four inches apart in front of the chest. Keep the fingers tensed.

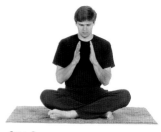

Step 3

3. Continue Long Deep Breathing for 1 minute as you hold the hands with palms facing each other in front of the chest and concentrate your gaze at the space between the palms. Keep the fingers tensed.

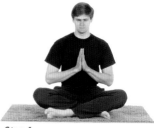

Step 4

4. Bring the hands with palms flat together, maintaining pressure and tension on the fingers as you continue Long Deep Breathing for 2 more minutes.

5. Now, keeping the hands with palms together in a prayer position, move the hands so they are in contact with the chest and press them against the center of the chest, which stills the mind, with normal breathing. Meditate in this position for 1 minute. Now relax the pressure on the hands. While concentrating at the third eye (a point of mental concentration that stimulates secretion of the pituitary gland, on the forehead slightly above where the root of the nose meets the eyebrows), slowly bend forward from the waist for 1 minute as you bring first the hands and then the forehead to the ground, bending forward. Meditate in this position for 1 minute. Then slowly come sitting back up over the next minute until you are again sitting in Easy Pose.

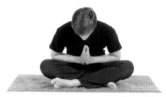

Step 5A

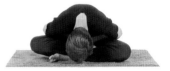

Step 5B

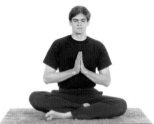

Step 5C

BENEFITS

One cycle of this meditation is also good as a preparation for meditation when you don't feel like meditating. It is said that this meditation burns off childhood fear blocks, phobias and negativity from your magnetic field if you practice this meditation forty times in a 24-hour period.

Total Time: 9 minutes

MEDITATION 7C MEDITATION FOR SUBCONSCIOUS TEMPERAMENTAL FEAR

There is a meditation (Meditation 7C) to help clear the subconscious mind of fear. Practice this meditation for at least the minimum time on a daily basis for forty days. Then evaluate how this meditation has changed your life.

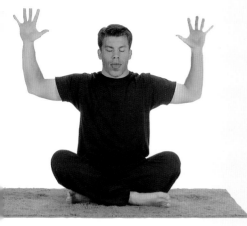

7C

Sit in Easy Pose with a straight spine. Bring the arms up 90 degrees out to sides, with forearms perpendicular to ground, fingers spread apart, palms facing forward. Chin in, chest out. Stick the tongue out all the way, and bite gently on it. Eyes open as slits. Slow Long Deep Breathing through the nose for 11 minutes. You can increase the time to 31 minutes over a period of ninety days of regular practice. The best mantra mentally with the breath is "Go" on inhale, "Bind" on exhale.

To end the meditation: Inhale and then exhale for a total of three times, then stretch spine and arms and shoulders, and relax.

BENEFITS
This meditation clears the subconscious mind of temperamental fear.
Total Time: 11–31 minutes

MEDITATION 7D ❖ CALL FOR HELP

When you are in trouble, call for help. Here is the yogi way of calling for help:

Sit in Easy Pose with a straight spine. With the head facing forward, bring the chin in towards the Adam's apple; this applies a pressure to the back of the neck and aligns the neck vertebrae so they are in line with the rest of the straight spine. This is called Neck Lock, and it regulates the flow of energy into the brain. Inhale deeply through the nose and chant aloud a long "Sat" (holding out the *a* vowel sound for the length of the exhale) and then a short "Naam" at the end (Fig. 7D). Then inhale again, and chant again. *Sat* means Truth and *Naam* means name (Identity); *Sat Naam* means: truth is my identity. Continue for at least 5 minutes, or as long as you need until you feel comforted.

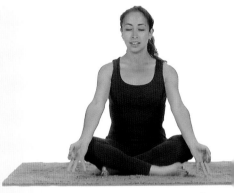

7D

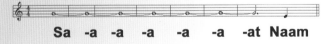

Sa -a -a -a   -a   -a   -at Naam

This is an example of how to vibrate the Cosmos (see sutra 5 in the final chapter of this book). It calls upon your inner essence and opens you up to new experience. You can relax because you call upon something greater than yourself for help. As Yogi Bhajan says, "The One who rotates the earth can take care of your routine."

BENEFITS

Prayer works, and this prayer is like a one-ounce key that can open up a sixty-pound lock. It is one of the most effective sounds you can create, and it has the power to open every door.

Total Time: 5 minutes or longer until you feel comforted

EXERCISE 7E ❖ CALMING HYSTERIA

Earlier in this book, I discussed how powerfully the breath affects the mind. Here is a useful technique for bringing someone who is hysterical back to normal consciousness within 3 minutes.

Get the person's attention and have them begin breathing one breath per minute in this manner: Inhale as slowly and deeply as possible through the nose for 30 seconds, then exhale slowly through the nose for 30 seconds. Continue for 3 minutes. By the time the person has completed three breaths, they will be back to normal.

BENEFITS
Relieve hysteria quickly.
Total Time: 3 minutes

CHAPTER EIGHT
Crisis Situations

Our world changed in September 2001 with the terrorist attacks on New York City and Washington, D.C.

The workplace and our fellow citizens are on alert, more cautious of our safety and environments than ever before. The natural tendency is to shut down from emotional overload, but instead, greater sensitivity and awareness is required. The Meditation for Hair Trigger Efficiency helps you to develop the ability to remain calm and alert in any crisis situation, so you can take care of business more effectively.

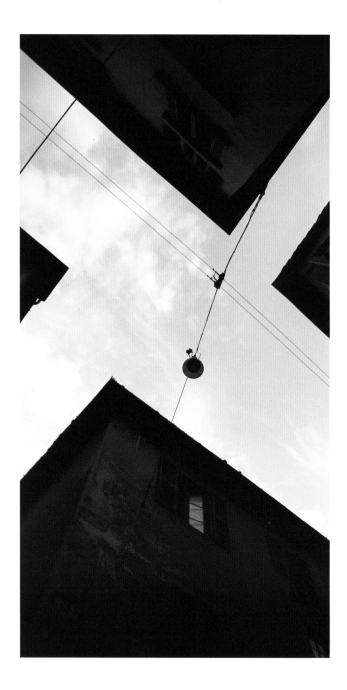

MEDITATION 8 ❖ FOR HAIR TRIGGER EFFICIENCY

Sit in Easy Pose with a straight spine. With the elbows bent, raise the hands up and in until they meet at the level of the heart a few inches from the body. With the fingers of both hands extended and joined, and the palms facing the body, place the palm of the right hand over the back of the left hand. The fingers of the left hand point toward the right and the fingers of the right hand point toward the left. Press the thumbtips together. Hold the hands and forearms parallel to the ground.

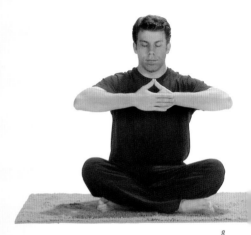

Keep the eyes one-tenth open. Inhale deeply through the nose and hold the breath for 10 seconds. Exhale completely through the nose and hold the breath out for 10 seconds. The air must go all the way

8

out on the exhale so that all the heart valves get equal pressure, and the brain and central nervous system will trigger survival mode for a few seconds. Continue this breathing pattern. Concentrate powerfully on the breath.

Practice this meditation 3 to 5 minutes at a time.

BENEFITS

This meditation brings the entire nervous and glandular system into balance. By putting the thumbs together in the mudra the sciatic nerve is neutralized at the point of ego. This particular balance puts pressure on certain meridian points in the shoulders.

In doing the meditation you will come to understand that even with the breath out you are still alive. A lot of prob-

lems in family and social relationships can occur if you do not have control over the breath. The beauty of life is based on the breath. It is the link between you and Infinity and it is what gives you the sensitivity to feel all around you.

Do this meditation at lunchtime or any time you want to get sharp and have an edge over another person. It can give you hair trigger efficiency in a life and death situation.

Total Time: 3–5 minutes

CHAPTER NINE

For Protection

Sometimes we need protection in grave or dangerous situations. The Guru Mantra (Meditation 9) can be chanted whenever you need protection or divine assistance.

I was driving with my brother-in-law (also a yoga teacher) on an uncrowded, four-lane undivided highway in western Washington on a clear winter day, when the weather suddenly changed, as it often does along the Pacific Northwest coast, and it began hailing intensely. We slowed down to about twenty-five miles per hour to keep good traction on the road as the accumulating slush began to make the road very slippery.

After a half hour, the weather cleared. There were vehicles that were far enough ahead of us not to be visible, but their passage had ploughed deep furrows in the slush, so we followed in their tracks. Feeling more comfortable with road conditions and clear weather, I began to speed up.

Suddenly as we rounded a curve in the road, I lost control of the vehicle and it began to slide sideways toward the steep embankment and ditch on the right side of the road. Everything seemed to occur in slow motion as we headed helplessly for the embankment, where the car would probably crash-land sideways or perhaps turn over. I hung onto the steering wheel and cried out the Guru Mantra, calling directly to Guru Ram Das to save us. We continued to slide forward in slow motion as the car hydroplaned toward the edge of the road, and then

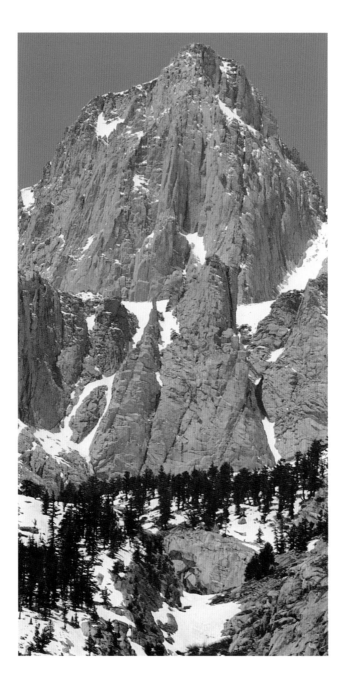

our trajectory changed as the car slid back toward the center of the road. The car spun to a sliding stop sideways across the center lines of the road and we were safe. My sense of time switched back to normal.

We looked at each other in astonishment and gratitude. The Guru had intervened. Then I quickly hit the gas pedal and got the car back onto our side of the road, and we were on our way again.

Establish a very personal relationship with your guru (or patron saint). You never know when you may need some divine intervention.

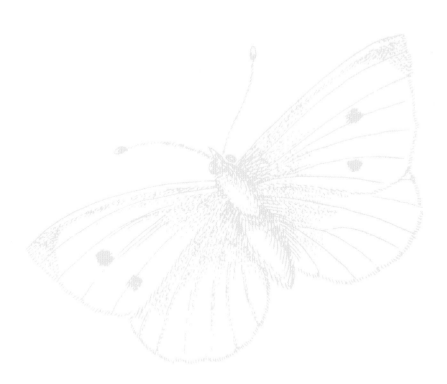

MEDITATION 9 ✣ GURU MANTRA

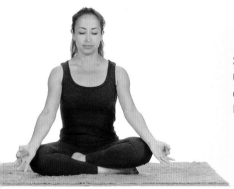

Sit in Easy Pose with a straight spine in Gyan Mudra. Rhythmically and melodiously chant the Guru Mantra for as long as you like:

Guroo Guroo Wah-hay Guroo
Guroo Raam Daas Guroo

BENEFITS

This meditation brings protection, relaxation, self-healing and emotional relief. This meditation can be useful, for example, at times when you are suffering the negative effects of office politics.

Total Time: 1 minute to 2½ hours

The mantra means "Wise, wise is the one who serves Infinity." The first phrase of this eight-beat mantra is a nirgun mantra (vibrates only to Infinity), and the second phrase is a sargun (finite form) mantra that connects the experience of Infinity to the finite. This meditation invokes the protective energy of Guru Ram Das, master of Kundalini Yoga and a great teacher and yogi of sixteenth-century India, by whose grace we today are able to practice the technology of Kundalini Yoga. This is a good meditation to practice whenever you need divine guidance, protection, or assistance. Miracles can happen.

CHAPTER TEN
Conquering Depression

The world is being transformed in the Information Age by new technologies that continue to emerge. Already knowledge workers are being overwhelmed by the sheer volume of information with which they must cope. When overwhelmed, people react by becoming stressed or chronically ill, with disrupted sleep cycles, behavioral addictions and compulsions, poor judgments and feelings of depression, helplessness, and withdrawal.[3]

Yogi Bhajan calls this malaise "cold depression." The World Health Organization has recognized that over the last twenty years, the incidence of depression has significantly increased[4] to become the number two killer in the world.[5]

In addition to the obvious effects of our rapidly evolving technology, humanity is also undergoing a significant evolutionary transformation: the transition into the Aquarian Age (year 2000 to year 3999), an era of increased brain power and mental sensitivity popularly known as an era of world peace and human brotherhood. According to Yogi Bhajan, the cusp period of this transition began in 1991 and will continue into the year 2012, by which time the Aquarian Age will be in full effect.

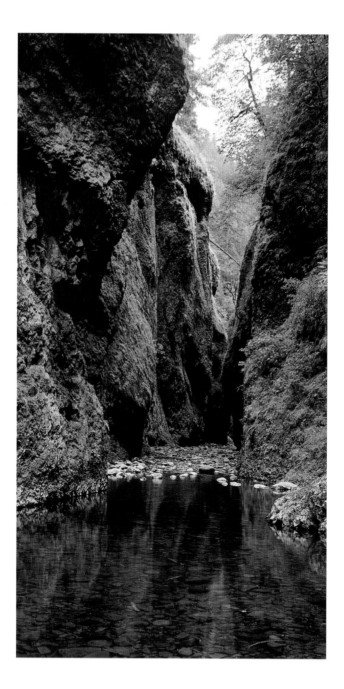

Yogi Bhajan describes the Aquarian Age as a sensitive mental era, where the technology of yoga/meditation will be much needed by humanity:

The human race is getting into a very sensitive mental era. . . .The new race which we are going to have on this planet will be the subject of some funny things, that is, that everybody will feel everything about everybody, and without figuring out why they feel or where they feel. But they feel. And this is going to make a person very crazy. . . . Unpredictable action of the human being will be the common trend in social living. . . . That shall be the coming race, because sensitivity in man's own self is going to increase, and mental mind projection is going to be very much activated, whereas the procedure to protect and channelize will be less known to people. . . . If your mind and your meditation and your sensitivity can be together [through the practice of yoga] . . . then you can be assured there will be a sensitive race anyway, but that race will sense everything clear, calm, and quiet. [6]

The high-touch technology that can save us from the distress caused by the high-tech[7] avalanche of information and the increasing but undisciplined mental sensitivity of the times is the science of yoga. The Meditation for Acute Depression is a good way to prevent and overcome the coming cold depression.

MEDITATION 10 ❧ HEALING MEDITATION FOR ACUTE DEPRESSION

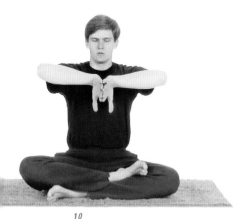

Sit in a comfortable meditative posture with a straight spine. Place the hands back to back with the fingers pointing away from the body at a level between the heart center and the throat center. Be sure that the knuckles touch. The wrists are about 6 inches away from the body. The forearms are as parallel to the ground as possible. The thumbs point straight down parallel to each other. This position creates a great deal of tension on the back part of the hand.

Eyes focus on the tip of the nose or on the upper lip. Inhale deeply and chant aloud "Wah-hay Guroo" sixteen times on the exhale. One complete cycle takes about 20 to 25 seconds.

10

Begin practice with 11 minutes. You may gradually increase the time to 31 minutes.

BENEFITS

This meditation can help begin to relieve the worst depression in just 11 minutes. When someone comes to you with a story of depression, don't get out of it by telling them you have your own problems. Instead, help them out of their depressed state with this meditation. That is one of the best ways to cure that emptiness within yourself.

Total Time: 11–31 minutes

CHAPTER ELEVEN
Anger Management

"Going postal" and "road rage" are recent additions to our cultural vocabulary that reflect the growing stress and frustrations of people at the beginning of the twenty-first century. As individuals under pressure we sometimes act impulsively impatient or intolerant; collectively, our behavior is gradually becoming more extreme with each passing decade.

Patience and tolerance are the direct results of having a strong nervous system. Unfortunately, many people do not yet know or practice yoga, one of the most effective technologies for strengthening the nervous system. Instead, Western civilization depends upon prescription drugs to control our mental states. There are tranquilizers, antidepressants, stimulants and more, with all their attendant deleterious side effects.

In contrast, yoga is a much more sophisticated approach. There are thousands of different yoga exercises and meditations, each designed to achieve a particular effect. Nothing external is required, no outside stimulus is needed to adjust the nervous system. The human already possesses from birth all of the equipment needed to do yoga.

The Meditation for Subconscious Temperamental Anger (Meditation 11) is a simple and easy meditation for resolving hidden or

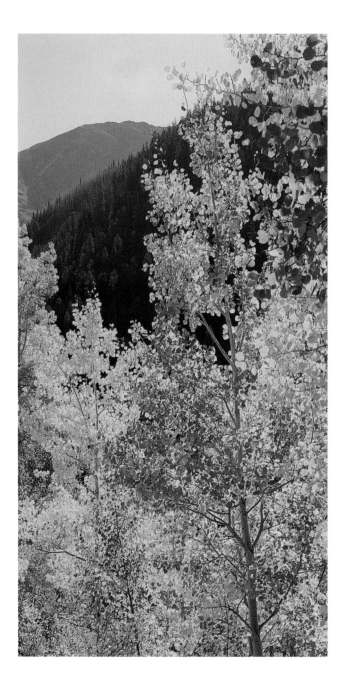

repressed anger. If you have issues with anger, try practicing this meditation for 11 minutes for ninety consecutive days.

At a recent reunion of my former employer, a longtime associate remarked that in all the years we had worked there, he had never seen me get angry and considers me unflappable. I am fortunate that over the years, besides doing this meditation, I followed the advice my yoga teacher once taught me—that you should carry anger in your pocket and only pull it out when you need it.

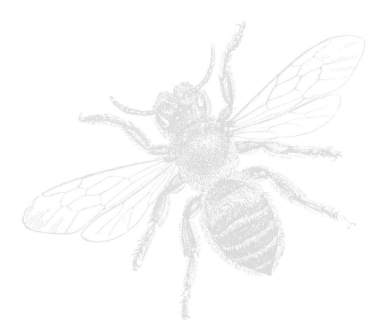

MEDITATION 11 ❁ MEDITATION FOR SUBCONSCIOUS TEMPERAMENTAL ANGER

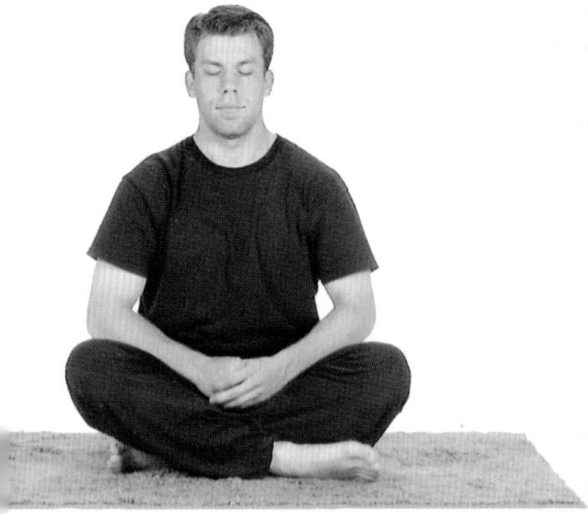

11

Sit in any pose, eyes open as slits; you can even do this meditation lying down. Hold the left thumb in the right fist, and enclose the right hand with the left hand, hands in lap. Meditate on the top of the head. Slow Long Deep Breathing through the nose for 11 minutes. You can gradually increase the time to 31 minutes over a period of ninety days' regular practice. The best mantra mentally with the breath is "Haring" repeated over and over. However, any of 2,000 different mantras can be used, including "Gobinday Mukanday Udaaray Apaaray Hareeang Kareeang Nirnaamay Akaamay"; "God and Me, Me and God are One"; or others.

The "r" sound in the mantra "Haring" is not mentally pronounced exactly like the normal American "r." If spoken aloud, this "r" would sound as if the tongue were flicking the upper palate in the same way it does making the "t" in the word "kitty."

You will want to do this meditation where others can't see you. It is a very private meditation.

BENEFITS

This meditation clears the subconscious mind of temperamental anger.

Total Time: 11–31 minutes

CHAPTER TWELVE

Clarity and Focus

Sometimes when our minds are clouded by doubt and indecision, we need clarity. The Meditation for Transformation (Meditation 12A) can help you clarify your direction in life and it enhances your communication. It improves self-image so your behavior can be in alignment with your self.

This meditation is one of several techniques given to help ease us into the twenty-first century. If you perfect this meditation, others can gain the benefits of it just by being in your presence.

For over twenty years, I told people that working with computers was my twentieth-century career, but teaching yoga was my twenty-first century career. During those two decades, I made a few unsuccessful efforts to teach yoga in the corporate environment where I worked every day. As an experiment in 1979, I taught a free midday yoga class at my workplace for over a month. It was enthusiastically received by employees, and one executive attended regularly; but, when I asked the company to pay for ongoing classes for employees, I was refused.

It was too difficult trying to integrate my two career interests, so I kept a low profile and assisted people on a personal basis—experiences that are the source of many of the anecdotes in this book.

In early 1999, I went through a critical period of doubt and confusion about what I should be doing with my life. I had been saying for

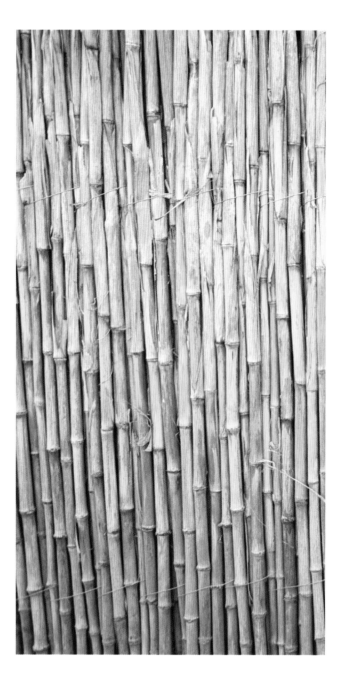

twenty years that I had a future yogic career, but had done nothing more than teach a weekly yoga class when I was not working day and night on projects for my employer.

I began practicing the Meditation for Transformation to clarify my life direction, eventually practicing for 31 minutes daily for 150 days. By the time that cycle was completed in late 1999, the Transition Stress Management business had been established and the first corporate classes taught. Shortly thereafter, I left employment in the computer field to focus full time on yoga and stress management consulting. My twenty-first-century career was launched.

MEDITATION 12A ❧ MEDITATION FOR TRANSFORMATION

Sit in a comfortable meditative posture with a straight spine.

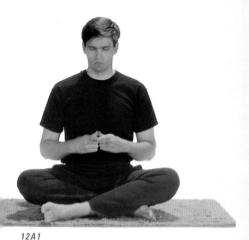

12A1

Place both hands in fists at the diaphragm. Touch the middle knuckles of each Saturn (middle) finger. Pressure on this central knuckle immediately gives self-confidence. Extend the Jupiter (index) fingers directly away from the body and let their end pads touch, forming a teepee. Extend the thumbs straight up and stretch them back as far as possible. They touch from the last knuckle to the tip (Figs. 12A1 and 12A3): their connection may be different with different people. If your ego is very large, they will not bend back very much and you will feel a lot of pain. Even if your ego is a little smaller and they bend back very far, the pain will still come after awhile.

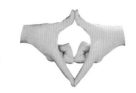

12A2

The hands are touching at the Saturn knuckles, Jupiter fingers, and thumbs. They are placed at the level of the diaphragm, touching the body. The thumbs are stretched back (Fig. 12A2).

Inhale deeply into the diaphragm and chant "Wah-hay Guroo" forty times on this one breath.

There are two important factors in this chant. First, when you run out of breath, stop. Do not cheat and continue chanting. Wait for the breath cycle to begin again. You may, however, begin by chanting "Wah-hay Guroo" sixteen or twenty-four times as you build up to forty repetitions, which is the ideal. Second, "Wah-hay Guroo" should be chanted in three parts. *Wah* means infinite; *Hay* means thou; and *Guroo* is the Self. When chanted in this manner, "Wah-hay Guroo" draws you very near to Infinity. So, there are three distinct parts to this meditation: *Wah, Hay,* and *Guroo.* They may be chanted slowly or not. The time doesn't really matter, but the three-beat rhythm does. It must be properly established.

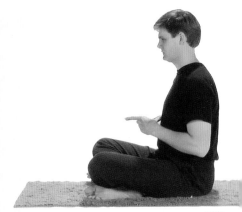

12A3

You may begin practice of this kriya with 10 to 15 minutes; there is no maximum limit, but 31 minutes is, generally speaking, a good length.

BENEFITS

When we see the dark clouds coming over the mountain, we seek shelter because we know there is an inherent danger in those clouds. We may get soaking wet; we may get struck by lightning. This meditation clears the darkness from the clouds in our hearts and helps us to avoid that inherent danger. It adjusts our perception of our projection and prevents weird actions resulting from a poor self-image.

To master this kriya, it must be practiced 120 days; that is, forty days for each of the three cycles. That is the shortest possible time. It may take as long as forty years. It depends on how vigorously and sincerely you practice it. However, you will almost always begin to notice some effects in about 120 days.

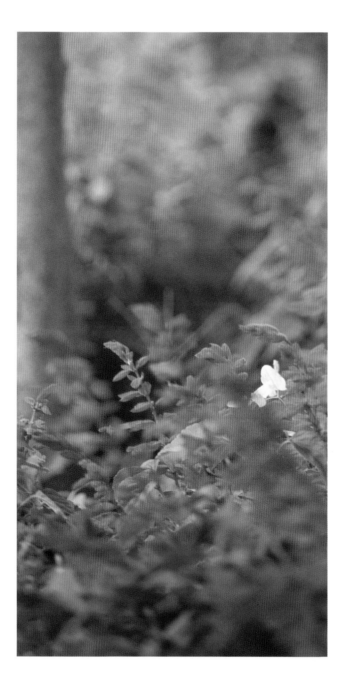

The effects are: 1) when you speak, the power of listening and understanding is automatically given to the person to whom you are speaking; 2) whatever you say, you shall remember; and 3) your sayings shall not be forgotten among humans.

Sometimes when you begin practice, you will feel a pressure around the lungs and the thyroid gland. This is a very temporary effect. Later you will feel very young, very energetic, and very levitated. The action of the tongue as it flicks the upper mouth causes the central nerve on its tip to be stimulated. This causes the thalamus to secrete and drip, the pineal to radiate, and the pituitary to secrete. The energy at your navel point will run down to the base of your spine, then back all the way up, back and forth. You will get a feeling of vast horizons; they call it enlightenment.

—Yogi Bhajan

Total Time: 10–31 minutes

MEDITATION 12B ❋ MEDITATION FOR CONCENTRATION IN ACTION

Some people cannot meditate because their physical condition prohibits sitting up straight, or their nervous system is so weak that they cannot focus or be still long enough to enjoy the benefits of meditation. The Meditation for Concentration in Action (Meditation 12B) is a meditation for people who are unable to meditate. It can calm the most fluctuating mind.

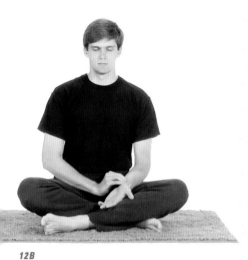

12B

Sit in a comfortable meditative posture with a straight spine. With the four fingers of the right hand, feel the pulse on the left wrist. Place the fingers in a straight line pressed lightly so that you can feel the pulse in each fingertip. Focus your mind at the point where the nose and eyebrows meet. The eyelids are lightly closed. On each beat of the heart, mentally hear the sound "Sat Naam."

Practice this for 11 minutes. Over a period of days or weeks, gradually increase the time to 31 minutes.

BENEFITS

If you don't know how to meditate or you want to develop this ability of concentration in action, there is a beautiful Kundalini Yoga technique to achieve it. This is a meditation for someone who can't meditate. It allows you to control your own reaction to any situation and can bring sweetness and onepointedness to the most outrageous and scattered mind.

Total Time: 11–31 minutes.

CHAPTER THIRTEEN

Improving Intuition

Over the years, I have relied a lot on intuition in the workplace. From selecting among well-qualified job candidates, to sensing the right moment to provide feedback, to sizing up business opportunities, intuition can be a deciding factor.

What is the right course of action to take in any given situation? This meditation enhances your intuition so your brain can instantly compute the correct action. It directly stimulates the pituitary gland, the master endocrine gland that regulates the entire glandular system.

One of the great things about this meditation is that it is the only meditation I know of that can be mastered in a short time, as little as one sitting. Most meditations can take months or years to master, depending upon the regularity and accuracy of your practice.

Mastery of a meditation means that the state of mind you are in during the meditation becomes immediately accessible to you, just by thinking about it. Imagine that you are practicing the meditation, and bingo—you are in that state of mind.

MEDITATION 13 ✤ DHRIB DHRISTI LOCHINA KARMA KRIYA

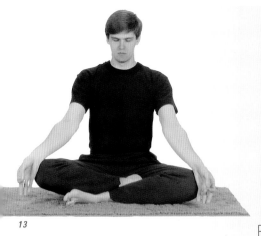

13

Sit in Easy Pose with a straight spine. The shoulders and hips should be in line. Now, lock the tips of the front teeth together. The eyes should look at the tip of the nose towards the chest. The tongue touches the upper palate (this should occur automatically within about 1 minute). Mentally project the mantra

Saa Taa Naa Maa

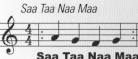

Saa Taa Naa Maa

out from the third eye. Beam it out, creating an internal harmony. Continue for 31 minutes.

BENEFITS

Dhrib Dhristi Lochina Karma Kriya is the "action of acquiring the insight of the future." This powerful yet simple meditation was first taught on the eve of a full moon. When practiced at this time, the effects are great as the subconscious mind is fully open to the vibratory action of the meditation. The pituitary gland is stimulated to secrete, which develops your intuition.

Although most meditations and kriyas require long periods of practice and mastery, it is possible to master this one in a single or several sittings. This is explained by the

wide range of individual differences between yoga practitioners and the uniqueness of this particular meditation. This meditation should be practiced for at least 31 minutes at a sitting. The minimum time is 15 minutes, and to master it you should practice for 1½ hours. Three hours' practice will open up the psychic capacities.

Total Time: 15–90 minutes

 Honestly practice this kriya and the following things will happen: Your eyes will have the power to heal anyone; your words will have the power to penetrate deeply; you will learn to talk inspiringly and your words will always represent the truth of a given situation (this is known as *vac siddhi*); you will be able to project your personality or your bodily sensations anywhere; and lastly, you will always know the consequence of any sequence that you may start.

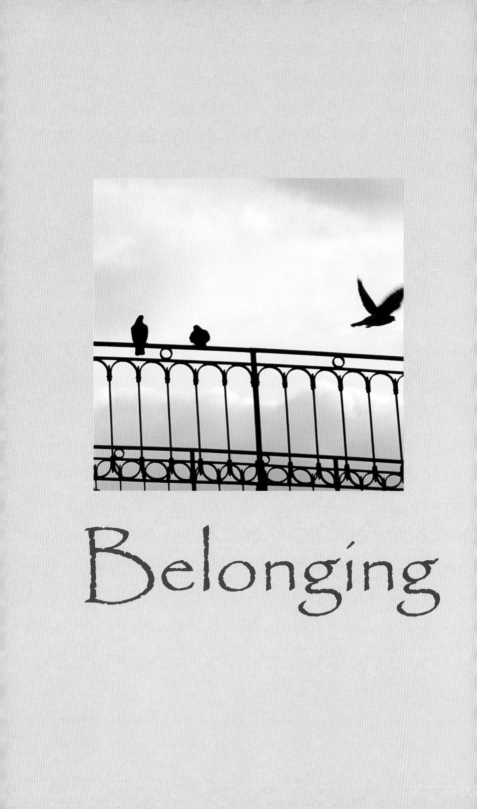

Belonging

CHAPTER FOURTEEN

Heart-Centered Management

Early in my business career I found that I could get things done by being focused and to the point, which was a comfort zone for my personality, but I was often so brusque and businesslike in the process that it hurt the feelings of my coworkers.

In an early position in my career, as manager of a group of a half dozen new associates, I managed to further alienate all of them by treating them as if they were equally qualified. Fortunately, the company offered a daylong course in management styles that allowed me to adjust the level and quality of supervision to match individual states of development. But the company at that time offered no training on interpersonal skills—how to interact without hurting others' feelings. Either you knew how to do that well, or you were not a manager for long. I learned by hard knocks and by practicing meditations for heart-centered awareness and neutral mind.

Personality traits, such as being an introverted overachiever, run deep into childhood and are difficult to modify. In all, it took me several years of effort in paying attention to others with a calm heart before I could act with confidence, knowing that my focus on business tasks and objectives would be, out of habit, balanced by sensitivity to the feelings of others. This is not to say that my behavior was always the best, but in general, I have been able to act with head and heart balanced.

Practicing the Meditation for a Calm Heart (Meditation 14) will help clarify your perception of others and give you the tranquility to act with sensitive awareness. This kind of subtlety is essential for leadership.

When your heart can't decide, use your head.
When your head can't decide, use your heart.

— Yogi Bhajan

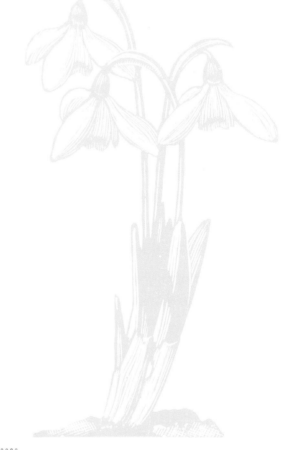

MEDITATION 14 ❖ MEDITATION FOR A CALM HEART

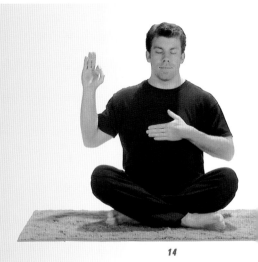

Sit in Easy Pose with a straight spine. Either close the eyes or look straight ahead with the eyes half open. Place the left hand on the center of the chest at the heart center level. The palm should be flat against the chest and the fingers parallel to the ground, pointing to the right. Make Gyan Mudra with the right hand by touching the tip of the index finger to the tip of the thumb. Raise the right hand up to the right side as if giving a pledge. The right palm faces forward and the three fingers not in Gyan Mudra point up. The right elbow is relaxed near the side with the forearm perpendicular to the ground.

14

Concentrate on the flow of the breath. Regulate each bit of the breath consciously. Inhale slowly and deeply through both nostrils. Then hold the breath in by suspending the chest. Retain it as long as possible. Then exhale smoothly, gradually, and completely. When the breath is totally out, lock the breath out for as long as possible. Continue this pattern of Long Deep Breathing with suspended inhalation and exhalation for 3 to 31 minutes. To end, inhale and exhale strongly three times and relax.

BENEFITS

The proper home of the subtle force known as *prana*, the life force that comes to you in the breath, is in the lungs and heart. The left palm is placed at the natural home of the prana. Create a deep stillness at that point. The right

hand that throws you into action and analysis is placed in a receptive, relaxed mudra and put in the position of peace. The entire posture induces a feeling of calmness. Technically, this meditation creates a still point for the prana at the heart center. Emotionally, this meditation adds clear perception to your relationships with yourself and others. If you were upset at work or in a personal relationship, sit in this meditation for 3 to 15 minutes before deciding how to act. Then act with your full heart. Physically, this meditation will strengthen the lungs and heart.

Total Time: 3–31 minutes

 This meditation is perfect for beginners. It opens your awareness of the breath and conditions your lungs. Try it for 3 minutes. If you have more time, try it for three periods of 3 minutes each with 1 minute rest between them, for a total of 11 minutes. When you hold the breath in or out for "as long as possible," you should not gasp or be under strain when you let the breath move again. For an advanced practice of concentration and rejuvenation, build the time of this meditation up to 31 minutes.

CHAPTER FIFTEEN

Relax and Rejoice

If my day at the office was particularly difficult or stressful, what I needed on arrival at home was some quick and effective R&R. Yogis do not drink alcohol or take intoxicants, but there are some excellent techniques for getting quick relaxation.

The Meditation to Relax and Rejoice (Meditation 15) is effective, so long as you don't have anything important to do or that requires concentration. Try a different meditation if you do, because this one could put you in orbit for the rest of the day.

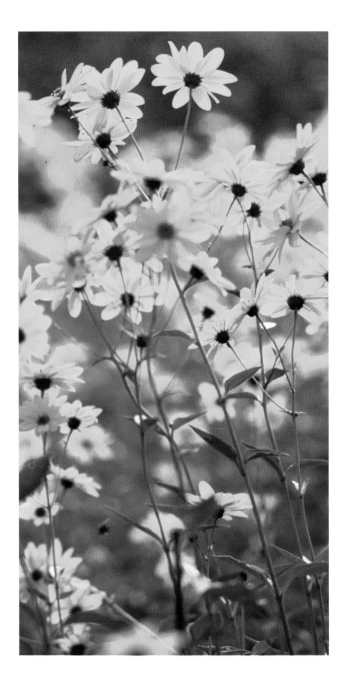

MEDITATION 15 ❖ MEDITATION TO RELAX AND REJOICE

Sit in Easy Pose with a straight spine, but be relaxed in the position. Relax the arms down by the sides of the body with the elbows bent. Draw the forearms in toward each other until the hands meet in front of the body. Make a fist of the left hand and stick the thumb down into the middle of the fist. Wrap the right hand around the left fist and place the right thumb over the left fist, on top of the base of the left thumb.

Focus the eyes on the tip of the nose. Deeply inhale through the nose, then completely exhale as you chant the following mantra in a monotone:

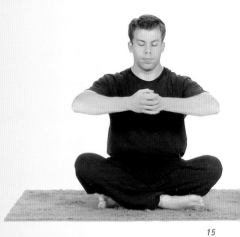

Haree Har, Haree Har,
Haree Har, Haree Har,
Haree Har, Haree Har,
Haree Har, Haree Har.

Begin by practicing the meditation for 10 to15 minutes and slowly build the time to 1 or 2 hours.

15

Har means the creative energy of the universe. The vowel sound in "Haree" and "Har" is a short a sounded like the word "the." The "r" sound in "Haree" and "Har" is not pronounced exactly like the normal American "r." While making this "r" sound, the tongue flicks the upper palate in the same way it does making the "t" in the word "kitty."

BENEFITS

This meditation is to help you relax and rejoice. It enables you to understand the contrast between working from

your ego and working from your inner self, the will of the Infinite, the soul.

Total Time: 10–62 minutes

 This is a very spacey meditation, so practice it when you have nothing to do for a while. This is not a meditation to practice if immediately afterwards you have to drive a car or perform other activities that require concentration.

CHAPTER SIXTEEN Happiness

If you think about the times in your life that you have been truly happy, can you identify any elements these times have in common?

For myself, some of the elements are love (the experience of selflessness within oneself), and being "in the flow" of whatever I am doing.

Here are "Seven Steps to Prosperity" that Yogi Bhajan has identified:

1. Commitment, is a must in a Human

2. Character, is the Glory of a Human

3. Dignity, is the Courage of a Human

4. Divinity, is the Strength of a Human—Physical & Mental

5. Grace, is all power of the Human

6. Power to Sacrifice, is *Dasvandh* (charity)—Giving is like God, His only act is Giving

7. Happiness, enjoy the ecstasy and exalted feeling of it all

MEDITATION 16 ❀ SMILING BUDDHA KRIYA

The Smiling Buddha Kriya (Meditation 16) will help you to experience happiness. The radiance you experience will enable you to uplift the hearts of others just by being in their presence.

Historically, this is a very outstanding kriya. It was practiced by both Buddha and Christ. The great brahman who taught Buddha this kriya found him in a nearly starved and unhappy condition. Buddha was unable to walk after his forty-day fast under the fig tree. He began eating slowly. That great brahman fed him and massaged him. When Buddha finally started smiling again, the brahman gave him this one kriya to practice.

Jesus also learned this meditation in his travels. It was the first of many that he practiced. You might begin to understand his state of consciousness by practicing what he practiced. You have probably seen this hand mudra or gesture in paintings and statues. It is a gesture and exercise of happiness and it opens the flow of the heart center.

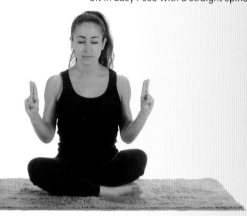

Sit in Easy Pose with a straight spine. With each hand, curl the ring and little fingers and press them down with the thumb, keeping the first two fingers straight. Bring the arms up so the elbows are pushed back and a 30-degree angle is made between the upper arm and forearm. The forearms must be parallel. The palms face forward. Make sure the elbows are pressed back and the chest is out (Figs. 16A1 and 16A2). Concentrate at the third eye very powerfully. Chant mentally at the point of the third eye:

16A1

Saa Taa Naa Maa.

Saa means Infinite, beginning.
Taa means Life, existence.
Naa means Death.
Maa means Rebirth, regeneration.

The whole mantra means "I am Truth."

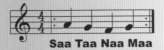

Saa Taa Naa Maa

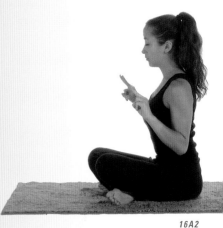

16A2

Do this for 11 minutes, then inhale deeply, exhale, open and close the fists several times, and relax.

BENEFITS

This meditation gives you the experience of happiness and compassion in a state of grace. Practice this meditation to be yourself and experience your higher consciousness. Master the technique and experience the state it brings, then share it by creating beauty and peace.

Total Time: 11 minutes

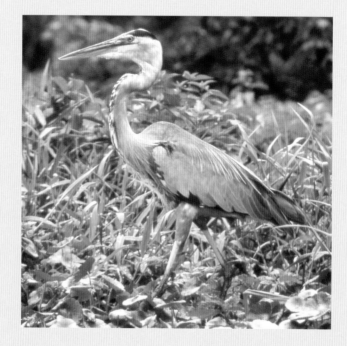

Self-
Esteem

CHAPTER SEVENTEEN

Perseverance

When your navel point is strong, it makes your communication direct and to the point, and it gives you the ability to see things through to completion. If your navel point is weak, you probably find it difficult to stay focused and to complete projects and tasks.

Each of the exercises in this chapter adjusts the entire nervous system as all 72,000 major nerves flow through the navel point and are coordinated there.

During the mid-1990s, I spent two years on the road on business. I worked at corporate client sites for three months at a time and had to live in hotel rooms. About once a month I traveled home for a weekend, then had to go back. It was a lonely time, and I had many responsibilities and much work to do. Every morning I practiced an hour-long Nabhi (navel strengthening) Kriya so that I could stay focused and complete my work. It was very helpful, and I am not sure how I could have endured and achieved success had I not practiced it. It was quite difficult, but it made the rest of my day look like a piece of cake!

Here are two simple exercises you can practice for 1 to 3 minutes daily, that will gradually develop your navel strength. Relax on your back for an equal amount of time after completing each exercise.

EXERCISE 17A ✤ STRETCH POSE

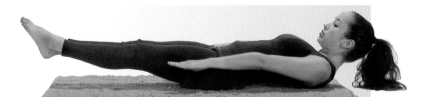

Lie on your back and come up into Stretch Pose (Fig. 17A): head and feet up six inches off the ground, balanced at the navel point, arms straight with fingers pointed toward the toes and palms down, and stare at the toes. Breath of Fire for 1 minute. Mentally inhale "Sat" and exhale "Naam" with each breath. This exercise moves your pulse directly under the navel to center the physical body. To end, inhale, then exhale and hold the position while squeezing Mool Bhand for a few seconds (contract the muscles of the rectum and sex organ and pull the navel in toward the spine), then relax on your back for at least 1 minute.

BENEFITS
Centers the physical body. Strengthens the nervous system.

Total Time: 2 minutes

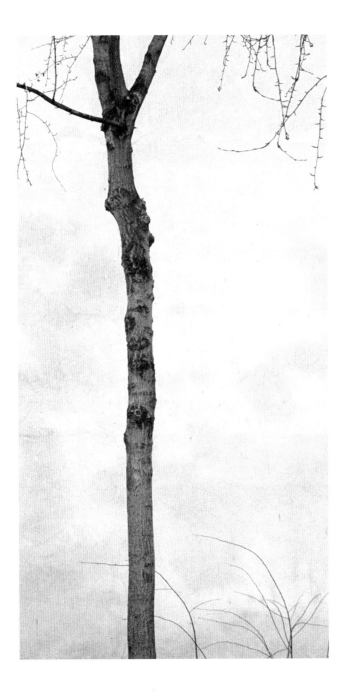

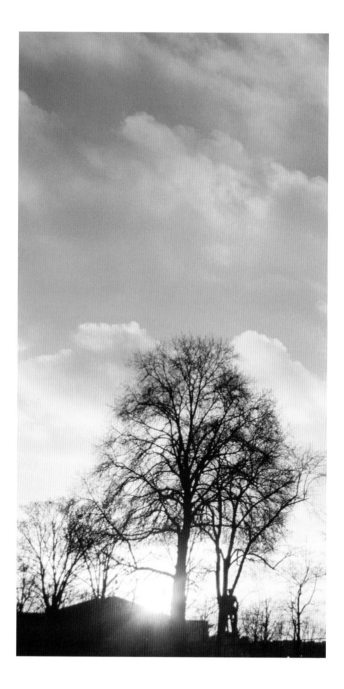

EXERCISE 17B ✥ MARTIAL ARTS NAVEL STRENGTHENING EXERCISE

This exercise is more powerful than Stretch Pose, so you should become proficient in practicing Stretch Pose before undertaking this exercise.

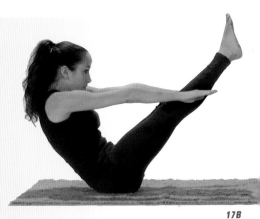

17B

Lie on your back and bring the torso to 60 degrees and the legs straight up to 60 degrees with the arms parallel to the ground with palms facing down (Fig. 17B). Breath of Fire for 1 minute. Concentrate at the navel point and mentally loudly inhale "Sat" and exhale "Naam" through the nose with each breath. This exercise strengthens the navel point. To end, inhale, then exhale and relax on the back for at least 1 minute.

BENEFITS

Strengthens the navel point. Strengthens the nervous system.

Total Time: 2 minutes

EXERCISE 17C ❧ NABHI KRIYA

Nabhi Kriya is a bit more strenuous. Try it if you are feeling adventurous.

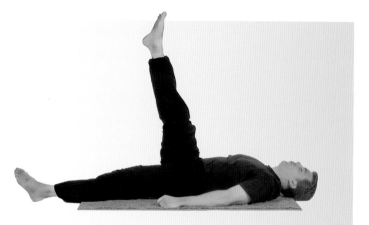

Step 1

1. Lie flat on the back. Inhale and lift the right leg up to 90 degrees, then exhale and let it down. Repeat with the opposite leg. Continue alternate leg lifts, keeping the breath through the nose deep and powerful for 10 minutes.

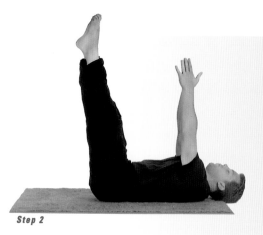

Step 2

2. Without stopping, begin to lift both legs up to 90 degrees with the inhale, and down with the exhale. Stretch the arms straight up toward the sky, palms toward each other. Keep the arms fixed for balance and energy. Continue for 5 minutes.

3. Pull the knees onto the chest. Hold them there with the arms. Let the head relax back. Rest in this position for 5 minutes.

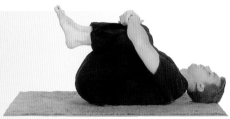

Step 3

4. Starting with the position in Step 3, inhale and extend the arms straight out from the sides on the ground, extending the legs straight to a 60-degree angle.

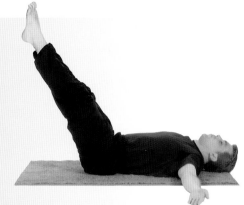

Step 4A

On the exhale, return to the original position. Continue for 15 minutes.

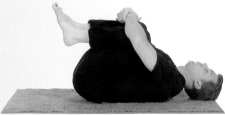

Step 4B

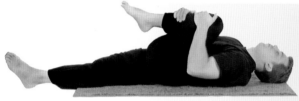

Step 5A

5. Lie on the back. Bring the left knee to the chest. Hold it there with both hands.

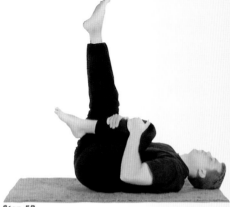

Step 5B

Begin rapidly lifting the right leg up to 90 degrees and down to the ground. Exhale as the leg goes down, inhale as it raises. Continue for 1 minute.

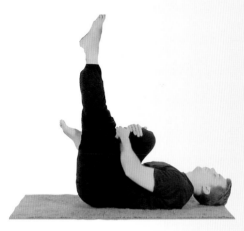

Step 5C

Then switch legs for 1 minute. Repeat the complete cycle for both legs one more time.

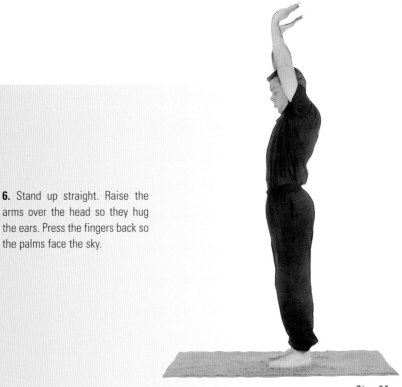

Step 6A

6. Stand up straight. Raise the arms over the head so they hug the ears. Press the fingers back so the palms face the sky.

Exhale and bend forward to touch the ground with the palms. While bending, keep the arms straight overhead and touching the ears. Inhale and raise up. Do this very slowly with a deep breath. On the exhale, apply Mool Bhand. Continue for 2 minutes, then increase the pace more rapidly for 1 more minute.

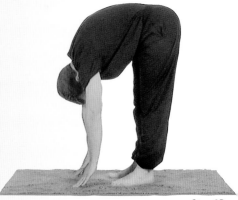

Step 6B

Step 7

7. Totally relax or meditate for 10 to 15 minutes.

BENEFITS

This set focuses on developing the strength of the navel point. The times indicated for each exercise are for advanced students. To begin the practice, start with 3 to 5 minutes on the longer exercises.

Step 1 is for the lower digestive areas. Step 2 is for the upper digestion and solar plexus. Step 3 eliminates gas and relaxes the heart. Step 4 charges the magnetic field and opens the navel center. Step 5 sets the hips and lower spine, and Step 6 is for the entire spine, spinal fluid, and the aura. Together, these exercises will get the abdominal area in shape very quickly.

Total Time: 29–57 minutes

CHAPTER EIGHTEEN

Breaking Bad Habits

You are the slave of your habits, but you can gradually substitute good habits for bad habits. Over a period of time, you will become a better person, and your life will be transformed.

Sam Pratt had a great sense of humor and he liked to joke with people around the office. Sam was attracted to women and could not resist verbalizing about their attributes to male coworkers when women were not around. One day he encountered an attractive female associate in the corridor just as she was coming out of the restroom. As it happened, she was adjusting her bra on the way out the door just as he walked up. "Need any help?" he asked in a humorous and friendly way. She filed a complaint of sexual harassment through the company's human resources department, and to resolve the situation without litigation, he resigned. A pretty powerful response to what he thought was his amusing sexual innuendo.

Although Sam was aware his off-color remarks were not appealing to women, his habit of joke-making overcame his better judgment. Too bad he did not know this technique for overcoming bad habits: the Meditation for Breaking Bad Habits (Meditation 18).

It takes forty days to establish a habit pattern. First you start the habit, then you are in the habit, and then you are the habit. It becomes part of your normal operating behavior.

Practice this meditation for 31 minutes every day for forty days. It will give you the ability to overcome seemingly unbreakable habits.

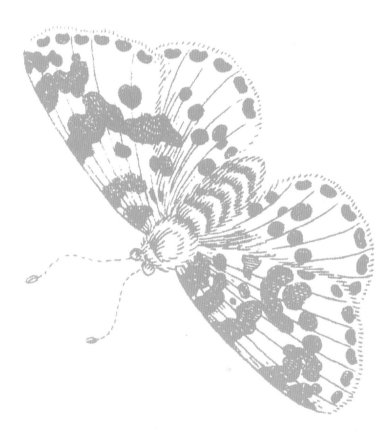

MEDITATION 18 ❖ MEDITATION FOR BREAKING BAD HABITS

Sit in a comfortable meditative posture. Straighten the spine and make sure the first six lower vertebrae are locked forward. Make fists of both hands and extend the thumbs straight. Place the thumbs on the temples and find the niche where the thumbs just fit. This is the lower anterior portion of the frontal bone above the temporal-sphenoidal suture.

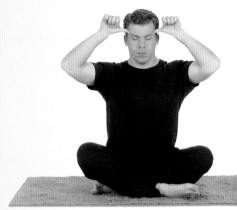

Lock the back molars together and keep the lips closed. Vibrate the jaw muscles by alternating the pressure on the molars. A muscle will move in rhythm under the thumbs. Feel it massage the thumbs and apply a firm pressure with the hands.

18

Keep the eyes closed and look toward the center of the eyes at the brow point. Silently vibrate the Panj Shabd mantra

Saa Taa Naa Maa

at the brow point in the same rhythm as the jaw muscles. Continue for 5 to 7 minutes. With practice the time can be increased to 20 minutes and ultimately to 31 minutes.

BENEFITS

The pressure exerted by the thumbs triggers a rhythmic reflex current into the central brain. This current activates the brain area directly underneath the stem of the

pineal gland. It is an imbalance in this area that makes mental and physical addictions seemingly unbreakable.

The imbalance in this pineal area upsets the radiance of the pineal gland itself, which in turn regulates the pituitary gland. Since the pituitary regulates the rest of the glandular system, the entire body and mind go out of balance. This meditation corrects the problem. It is excellent for everyone but particularly effective for rehabilitation efforts in drug dependence, mental illness, and phobic conditions.

Total Time: 5–31 minutes

CHAPTER NINETEEN

Good Decision Making

In business, as in other walks of life, you must be able to make good decisions.

Yogis have long recognized that the best decision making takes place when the left and right hemispheres of the brain are balanced and synchronized. Since the left brain questions and the right brain accepts, an individual's analytical and creative thought processes are most effective when a state of balance in neutrality is achieved. Yoga and meditation are effective technology for clearing the clutter of the mind's incessant chatter to reach a state of inner quietude where intuition flows and the solutions to even the toughest problems can be discovered.

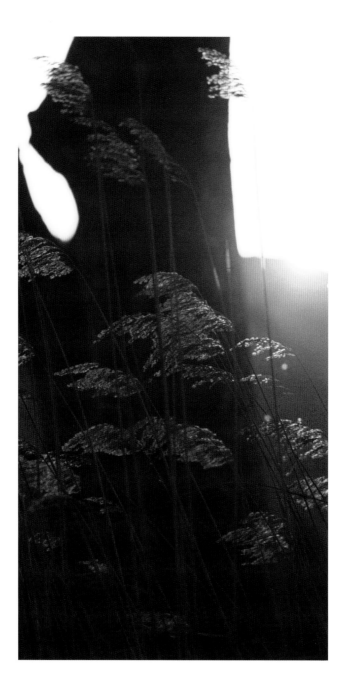

MEDITATION 19 ❖ TATTVA BALANCE
BEYOND STRESS AND DUALITY

This meditation balances the brain and relieves stress. It takes only 3 minutes but can have a profound effect.

Sit in Easy Pose with a straight spine. Raise the arms with the elbows bent until the hands meet at the level of the heart in front of the chest. The forearms make a straight line parallel to the ground. Spread the fingers of both hands. Touch the fingertips and thumb tips of opposite hands together. Create enough pressure to join the first segments (counting from the tip) of each finger. The thumbs are stretched back and point toward the torso. The fingers are bent slightly due to the pressure. The palms are separated. Fix your eyes at the tip of the nose.

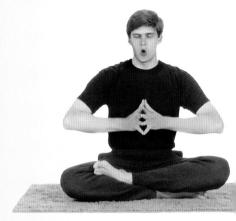

19

Create this breath pattern:

Inhale smoothly and deeply through the nose.

Exhale through the rounded lips in eight equal, emphatic strokes.

On each exhale pull the navel point in sharply. Continue for 3 minutes. Then inhale deeply, hold for 10 to 30 seconds, then exhale. Inhale again and shake the hands, then relax.

BENEFITS

The five *tattvas,* or elements (fire, air, water, earth, and ether), are categories of quality that are based in the

energetic flow of your life force. If all the elements are strong, in balance, and are located in their proper areas of the body, then you can resist stress, trauma, and illness. You also do not get confused in conflicts between the two hemispheres of the brain as they compete for the right to make and direct decisions.

Total Time: Three minutes. Build the practice slowly to 11 minutes. A longer duration is only for dedicated serious practitioners.

 This meditation uses the hand mudra to pressure the ten radiance points in the fingers that correlate to the zones of the brain in the two hemispheres. The equal pressure causes a kind of communication and coordination between the two hemispheres of the brain. The deep inhale gives endurance and calmness. The exhale through the mouth strengthens the parasympathetic system from a control band of reflexes in the ring of the throat. This calms reactions to stress. The strokes of the exhale stimulate the pituitary to assess the pressure and the balance, and to optimize clarity, intuition, and decision capacities. It resolves many inner conflicts, especially when the conflicts are from different levels of your functioning: spiritual vs. mental vs. physical or survival needs.

CHAPTER TWENTY

Charisma

The human magnetic field is the secret of all human interaction.

What do we mean when we say that someone has charisma? My *Webster's Dictionary* lists as one of the definitions of the word *charisma*: "a special magnetic charm or appeal of a person."

Just as an iron magnet has a magnetic field that surrounds it but is not visible to the naked eye, so the human body, which is ever so much more sophisticated than a lump of iron, has an invisible electromagnetic field that surrounds it. Modern science understands that the human nervous system runs on chemically induced electricity, and where there is electricity, there are electromagnetic fields. However, modern science (with the possible exception of Kirlian photography) has yet to measure and understand this phenomenon.

Some rare individuals have been able to see the human magnetic field, also known as the aura. The Meditation to Feel and See Your Energy Body (Meditation 20) can help you to experience this. It is not something mysterious that cannot be understood. With a little effort, you can experience your own magnetic field.

According to the yogis, the minimum animal aura extends out three feet from the physical body in all directions. The minimum human aura extends out seven feet beyond the physical body. Regular practice of yoga can strengthen and extend your aura at the rate of about one foot per year. When your *circumvent force* (one layer of the aura) is

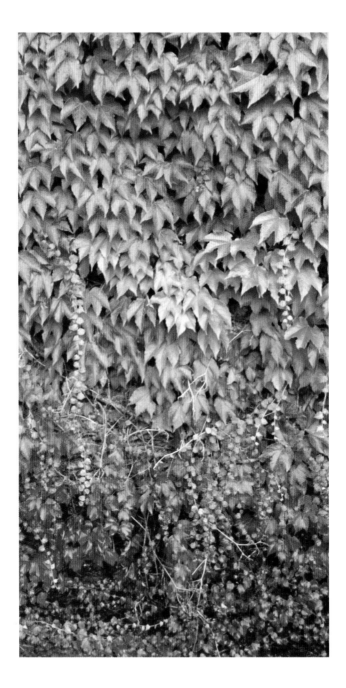

strong, negativity and negative circumstances are deflected away from you.

This means that two people typically begin interacting magnetically with each other at a distance of about fourteen feet. Sometimes you may meet people with whom you feel immediate like or dislike; this is an effect of the interaction between your magnetic fields. Your magnetic field carries the energy of all your previous thoughts, feelings and actions, so you always carry your baggage—and your dreams—with you.

Yoga and meditation can help lighten your load. By developing and strengthening your magnetic field, you can increase your radiance and positive effect upon others without conscious action, and generate healing energy.

I always found this magnetic effect to be beneficial in the work environment. People have told me they feel calmer in my presence. It has been a positive leadership quality.

MEDITATION 20 ❖ MEDITATION TO FEEL AND SEE YOUR ENERGY BODY

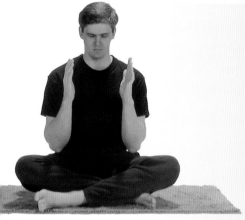

20

Sit in Easy Pose with your spine perfectly straight. Hold your upper arms near the sides of the chest. The forearms are 30 degrees out from the chest with the palms open and facing each other. The fingers are slightly spread and lightly cupped. Breathe long, deeply and slowly through the nose. Keep the eyes half open and focus between the palms.

As you breathe, feel the energy flow from one hand to the other. After a few minutes, you will begin to see the flow of energy. Do this for 11 minutes.

BENEFITS

This meditation gives you the ability to feel and see your energy body. It can make you aware of the potential conscious use of your electromagnetic field and of your subtle bodies as well as your physical body. It provides simple and direct experience of your magnetic field, which is a way of exercising a muscle you did not know you had that grows stronger over time.

Total Time: 11 minutes

CHAPTER TWENTY-ONE
Effective Communication

In business, and in every other domain of life, we can make or mar our success by how we communicate.

In order for your communication to be understood by another person, you must communicate on their frequency, and your words must penetrate to the heart of the person. Your whole being must be behind what you communicate or your communication will not be effective.

The Meditation for Effective Communication (Meditation 21) will help you develop the ability to communicate clearly.

Mostly our communication is trivial and mundane, or is intended to manipulate others. But if you speak nonsense, trivia, or untruths, the net result is that you confuse your own mind. So do not mar your success. Remember that in every communication with someone, you have a message to deliver. Be conscious that your communication is truthful, clear, and uplifting. You will be respected and loved, and your positive reputation will precede you.

Where the Infinite lives in you is on the tip of your tongue. Therefore, be careful that your words are kind, truthful, correct, and direct.

— Yogi Bhajan

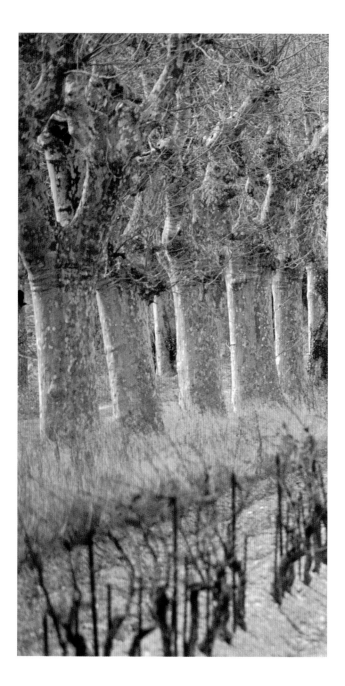

MEDITATION 21 ❖ KRIYA FOR EFFECTIVE COMMUNICATION

Sit in Easy Pose with a straight spine, or sit on a chair with feet on the ground and weight equally distributed on the feet. Interlock the hands and fingers with the right index finger on top of the left index finger and the thumbs joined and pointing straight up. Hold the hand position in front of the chest between the solar plexus and the heart. Relax the arms down with the elbows bent and the forearms pulled up and in toward the chest until the hands have met between the levels of the solar plexus and the heart (Figs. 21A1 and 21A2). Eyes are closed. Concentrate on the breath and the chanted mantra.

Deeply inhale through the nose and chant the mantra on the full exhale:

Raa Raa Raa Raa
Maa Maa Maa Maa
Saa Saa Saa Sat
Haree Har Haree Har

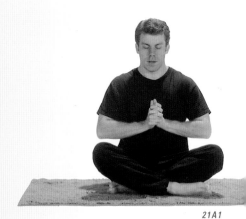

21A1

21A2

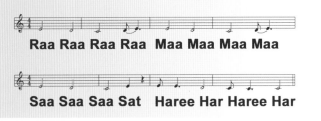

Raa Raa Raa Raa   Maa Maa Maa Maa

Saa Saa Saa Sat   Haree Har Haree Har

Be sure to chant the entire mantra with one full exhalation. Practice this meditation on an empty stomach. Practice this exercise for 15 minutes. Then end with a deep inhale; suspend the breath at least 15 seconds. Exhale through the mouth. Repeat three times. As a personal practice you can extend the time to 31 or 62 minutes, or longer. There is no time restriction on practice of this meditation.

The "r" sounds in this mantra are not pronounced exactly like the normal American "r." While making this "r" sound, the tongue flicks the upper palate in the same way it does making the "t" in the word "kitty."

Raa *is the father energy of the universe.* Maa *is the mother energy of the universe.* Sat *means truth.* Haree *is the creative energy of the universe. Together these sounds tune you into the creative essence within yourself.*

BENEFITS

This meditation will make your language very effective; so effective that you will not need to speak much to be heard.

Total Time: 15–62 minutes or more

This kriya gives you *gupt gyan shakti*, the secret knowledge of the power of your word to penetrate. Your power to penetrate depends on using the navel energy well. It also depends on your mental focus. Develop the habit in your communication of being conscious, with the full weight of your being behind what you speak. If you speak with awareness and clear intent, that aligns you with the subtle pulse of your being and its sound current.

CHAPTER TWENTYTWO

Prosperity

One of the best techniques I have used over the years to open up new avenues of opportunity is the Survasod ("Corrects Everything") Meditation. Among other things, it is good for self-healing, and for helping others with mental problems.

I used to teach a yoga class two evenings a week for psychiatric patients at a halfway house in Beverly Hills, California. Participants included manic-depressives, schizophrenics, psychedelic drug cases, paranoids, and other patients, and at the beginning they were all heavily medicated. To keep from going a little nuts myself while immersed in their unbalanced mental energy, I used to practice the Survasod Meditation before going there to teach.

One thing I noticed was that these students were very physically unbalanced. For example, one student could raise his right arm high up, but not his left arm; he was simply too stiff on one side. As they practiced yoga over a period of weeks and months, they began to develop more equal physical flexibility, and as they did so, they also became more mentally balanced. It was an amazing process to witness. The students who participated in yoga classes regularly were able to eliminate the need for medication, and some of them graduated out of the facility back to normal lives.

Over the years I often shared this meditation with interested coworkers who desired greater prosperity. This meditation surrounds you with healing green energy, and money is just "green energy." My observation has been that this meditation seems to open doors of opportunity to increase earnings. Let me know how it works out for you.

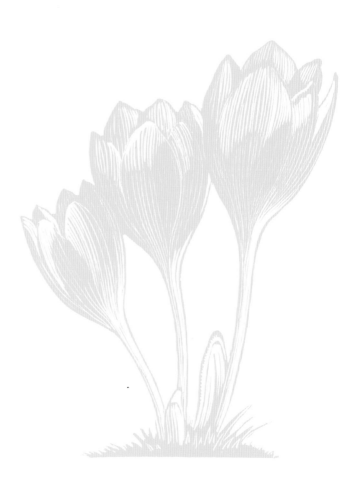

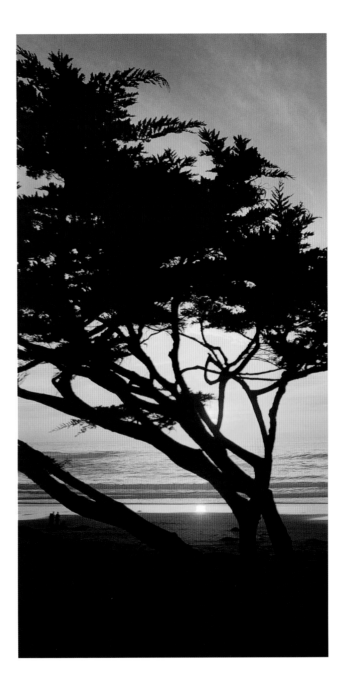

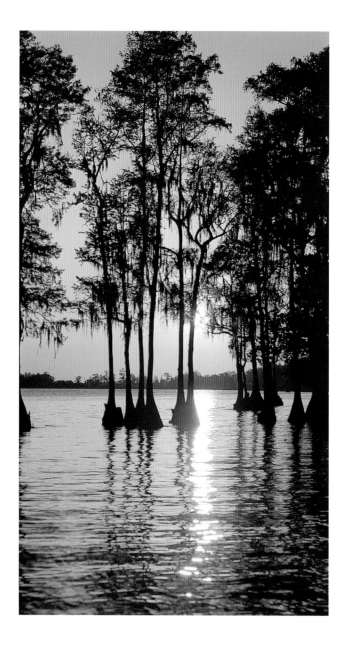

Yoga Secrets for Business Sucess

MEDITATION 22 ❖ SURVASOD MEDITATION

Sit in Easy Pose with a straight spine. First loosen and twist the spine from side to side. Lay right hand palm up on top of left hand palm up, thumbs touching. Palms are flat, facing up. Place hands against chest at diaphragm level. Concentrate at the brow point, slightly above where the root of the nose meets the eyebrows, with eyes closed, seeing the divine color green, the color of life.

Inhale deeply through the nose, and chant in a melody using the full breath:

Ha Ree, Ha Ree,
Ha Ree, Ha Ree,
Ha Ree, Ha Ree, Har.

22

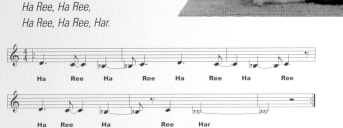

Then inhale and continue chanting the mantra once on each breath. The inhale is the eighth beat. Continue for 15 minutes. To end the meditation, inhale and hold the breath for a while, then exhale. Repeat the inhale and hold and exhale two more times.

The chanting is done long and slowly, and the melody is similar to "Saa Taa Naa Maa" (Kirtan Kriya) when sung. Har is the creative energy of the universe. The Ha is a short "a" as in "the," not long "a" ("Har" pro-

*nounced with a long a means destructive energy). The "Ha" and "Ree"
are separate sounds, not run together as one word, "Haree."*

*The "r" sound in this mantra is not pronounced exactly like the nor-
mal American "r." While making this "r" sound, the tongue flicks the
upper palate in the same way it does making the "t" in the word "kitty."*

BENEFITS

**Survasod is the "corrects everything" meditation. It is for
those who want to practice self-healing, and who want to
help others with mental problems. It is good for relationships, and increases lung capacity. It is commonly given
to students who want to get into the beauty of full-life
green energy; divine green energy will come to their
house. Worldly things will come and lift your spirit.**

Total Time: 15 minutes

CHAPTER TWENTYTHREE
Majesty of Self-Worth

Honestly answer the following questions, and write out your answers in longhand. Shut yourself up in a private place without interruptions and allow at least two hours to answer the following questions about yourself:

1. Describe your good points.

2. Describe your bad points.

3. Describe how you will overcome your bad points.

I always recommend undertaking this assignment to anyone who has problems with self-esteem. Do not show what you write to anyone, but do act upon what you discover. The results will astonish you.

The Sat Narayan Meditation (Meditation 23) is one of my personal favorite meditations of all time. No matter how miserable you may feel, this meditation will make you feel great. It makes your mind transparent so you can see clear through to the Infinity within you.

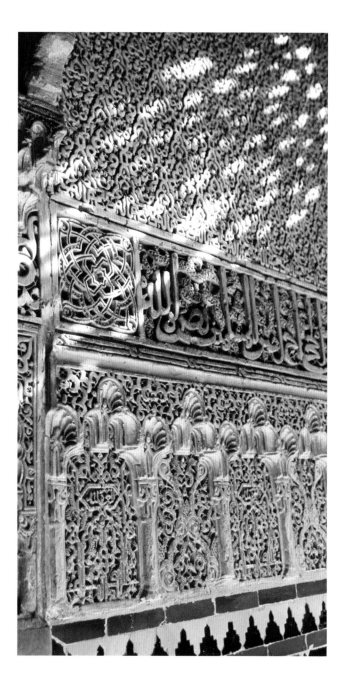

MEDITATION 23 ❖ SAT NARAYAN MEDITATION

Sit in Easy Pose with a straight spine. Bend the elbows at the sides, so the hands come up to about chin level. The hands are in Gyan Mudra, with the palms facing forward. The eyes are nine-tenths closed.

The mantra is

Sat Narayan Wah-hay Guroo
Haree Narayan Sat Naam

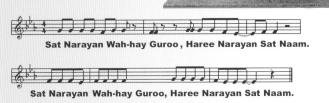

23

Sat Narayan Wah-hay Guroo , Haree Narayan Sat Naam.

Sat Narayan Wah-hay Guroo, Haree Narayan Sat Naam.

chanted in the melody above or in a monotone. It is chanted continuously, taking breath as needed.

Narayan *is the aspect of Infinity that relates to water.* Haree Narayan *is Creative Sustenance, which makes the one who chants it intuitively clear and healing.* Sat Narayan *is the True Sustainer.* Wah-hay Guroo *is indescribable Wisdom.* Sat Naam *means truth.*
The "r" sounds in this mantra are not pronounced exactly like the normal American "r." While making these "r" sounds, the tongue flicks the upper palate in the same way it does making the "t" in the word "kitty."

BENEFIT

Even the most lowly person, who feels like they have nothing or that they are nothing, can become completely majestic by chanting this mantra. It develops clarity of mind.

Total Time: 11–31 minutes

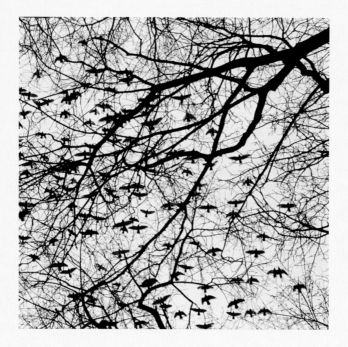

Self-
Realization

CHAPTER TWENTYFOUR
Cleansing the Subconscious

When the subconscious is clean, the conscious meets and merges with the subconscious, and they become the superconscious.

Kirtan Kriya (Meditation 24) is an incredible jewel, and a very powerful method for cleansing the subconscious mind. As you sit and do the meditation, all the hidden, suppressed garbage in your mind comes to the surface of your consciousness. As it does, you continue reciting the mantra to neutralize the effect of those thoughts.

Of all the meditations I have shared with people in the business environment over the years, this is the meditation I shared most frequently. It enables people to express themselves genuinely and fully. It lightens the load of your personality. It is effective and very healing.

Here Yogi Bhajan explains the importance of cleansing the subconscious mind:

A normal, fully aware human being has a mind that is stable, accurate, and neutral. Today most people are erratic, commotional, and upset by the smallest thing. Actually, nothing should upset you. You are beautiful. What upsets you is your own mind. It is the ugly mind that makes you think you are ugly. In fact, there is no such thing as an ugly human nature. It doesn't exist.

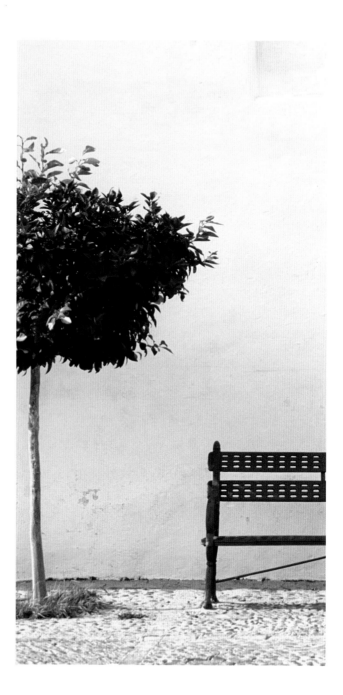

When the mind supports the thought pattern that you are ugly, then it can put you under a deep spell of self-delusion and depression. Under that spell, you can do undesirable and destructive actions. Your mind can drag you to the lowest level of your consciousness . . .

The mind must be able to know what it perceives and not confuse what it sees with its own subconscious projections. A huge amount of pain in human life comes from treating something not as it really is, but as you project it is. This creates confusion and delusion . . .

You project yourself and create a role, with its commitments, when you speak and give your word. Your mind must be taught to listen to your word, to see clearly what you have created and to live to that word in activity. No one should forget this.

Your projected personality in activity is what you are. How you act in relation to another person is what matters. All scriptures talk about it.

Whether you have money or you don't; whether you are healthy or unhealthy; or whether you are a good person or a bad person doesn't matter at all. It is not your initial status in life, but your habit in personality that matters. It is how you project yourself in activity, for that will create your reality, your impact, and your future. [8]

MEDITATION 24 ❖ KIRTAN KRIYA

Sit in Easy Pose with a straight spine. Meditate at the brow point and utter the five primal sounds (Fig. 24A), known as the Panj Shabd: S, T,

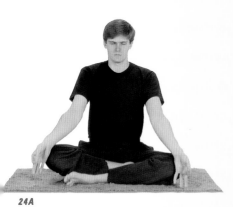

N, M, A. These five sounds are combined into four syllables of the mantra Saa Taa Naa Maa that is recited repeatedly throughout the kriya. Their meaning is:

> *Saa: means Infinite, beginning.*
> *Taa: means Life, existence.*
> *Naa: means Death.*
> *Maa: means Rebirth, regeneration.*

This is the cycle of creation. From the infinite comes life and individual existence. From life comes death or change. From death comes the rebirth of consciousness to the joy of the infinite through which compassion leads back to life. This sound current is represented musically this way:

24A

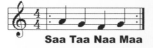

Saa Taa Naa Maa

Each repetition of the entire mantra takes 3 to 4 seconds.

The elbows are straight while chanting, and each fingertip touches in turn the tip of the thumb with firm pressure. The proper sequence of hand positions (mudras) in this meditation is illustrated in Figures 24B, 24C, 24D and 24E.

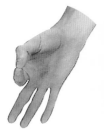

MUDRA 24B
On "Saa" touch the first, the Jupiter finger, to the thumb.

24B

MUDRA 24C

On "Taa" touch the second, the Saturn finger, to the thumb.

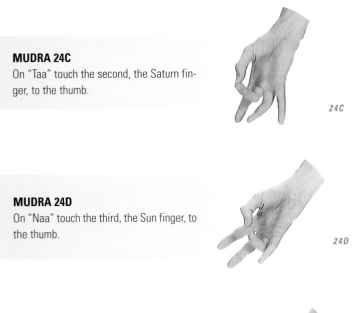

24C

MUDRA 24D

On "Naa" touch the third, the Sun finger, to the thumb.

24D

MUDRA 24E

On "Maa" touch the fourth, the Mercury finger, to the thumb.

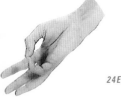

24E

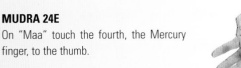

Then begin again on the first finger (Mudra 24B).

Chant in the three languages of consciousness:

> *Human: things, the world; normal or loud voice*
> *Lovers: longing to belong; strong whisper*
> *Divine : infinity; mentally (silent)*

Begin the kriya in a normal voice for 5 minutes, then whisper for 5 minutes, and then go deep into the sound silently. Vibrate in silence for 10 minutes, then come back to a whisper for 5 minutes, then aloud for 5 minutes. You may adjust the length of the meditation for more or less than 30 minutes, but keep each voice sequence the same length; for example, to practice this meditation for 18 minutes, keep each

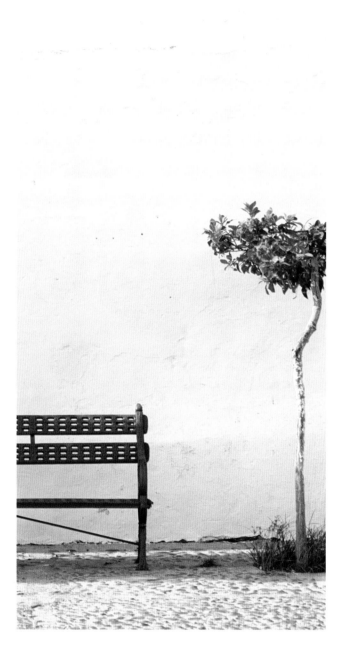

voice sequence to 3 minutes: aloud 3 minutes, whisper 3 minutes, silent 3 minutes, silent 3 more minutes, whisper 3 minutes, aloud 3 minutes.

To end, inhale and exhale. To come completely out of the meditation, stretch the hands up as far as possible and spread them wide. Stretch the spine and take several deep breaths. Relax.

Each time you close a mudra by joining the thumb with a finger, your ego "seals" the effect of that mudra in your consciousness. The effects are as follows:

SIGN	FINGER	NAME	EFFECT
♃	1ST, Jupiter	Gyan Mudra	*Knowledge*
♄	2ND, Saturn	Shuni Mudra	*Wisdom, intelligence, patience*
☀	3RD, Sun	Surya Mudra	*Vitality, energy of life*
☿	4TH, Mercury	Bhuddi Mudra	*Ability to communicate*

Practicing this chant brings a total mental balance to the individual psyche. As you vibrate on each fingertip, you alternate your electrical polarities. The index and ring fingers are electrically negative, relative to the other fingers. This causes a balance in the electromagnetic projection of the aura.

If during the silent part of the meditation your mind wanders uncontrollably, go back to a whisper, to a loud voice, to a whisper, and back into silence. Do this as often as needed.

Practicing this meditation is both a science and an art: It is an art in the way it molds consciousness and in the refinement of sensation and insight it produces; it is a science in the tested certainty of the results each technique produces. Meditations have coded actions to their reactions in the psyche. But because it is effective and exact it can also lead to problems if not done properly.

Some people may experience headaches from practicing Kirtan Kriya. The most common reason for this is improper circulation of prana in the solar centers. To avoid this problem or correct it if it has already occurred, you must meditate on the primal sounds in the "L" form. This means that when you meditate you feel there is a constant inflow of cosmic energy into your solar center, or tenth gate at the top of the head. As the energy enters the top chakra, you place "Saa," "Taa," "Naa," or "Maa" there. As you chant "Saa," for example, the S starts at the top of your head and the A ends through the brow point as it is projected to infinity. This energy flow follows the energy pathway called the golden cord—the connection between the pineal and pituitary glands.

Chanting "Saa Taa Naa Maa" is the primal or nuclear form of "Sat Naam." It has the energy of the atom in it since we are breaking the atom (or beej) of the sound, "Sat Naam."

You may use this chant in any position as long as you adhere to the following requirements:

1. Keep the spine straight.
2. Focus at the brow point.
3. Use the L form of meditation.
4. Vibrate the Panj Shabd in all three languages.
5. Use yogic common sense without fanaticism.

BENEFITS

This meditation cleans the subconscious mind. It enables a person to be forthright, direct, and sincere in thought, word, and action. It makes you authentically you.

Total Time: 31 minutes

At the winter solstice of 1972, Yogi Bhajan said that a person who wears pure white and meditates on this sound current for 2½ hours a day for one year will know the unknowable and see the unseeable. Through this constant practice, the mind awakens to the infinite capacity of the soul for sacrifice, service, and creation.

CHAPTER TWENTY-FIVE
Manifesting Your Potential

One of the most effective techniques for purifying and elevating your consciousness is the Sat Kriya exercise. Yogi Bhajan has recommended that if you do no other yoga exercise regularly, you should do Sat Kriya (Exercise 25) for up to 31 minutes a day: "You must grind yourself to know your grounds."

As a beginner, 3 minutes' practice is the recommended duration. You can gradually extend the time of each session by 1 minute or so over a period of weeks as you develop the nerve strength and stamina to do more. Enjoy the gradual unfolding of expanded consciousness as you slowly and steadily develop your capacity for greatness.

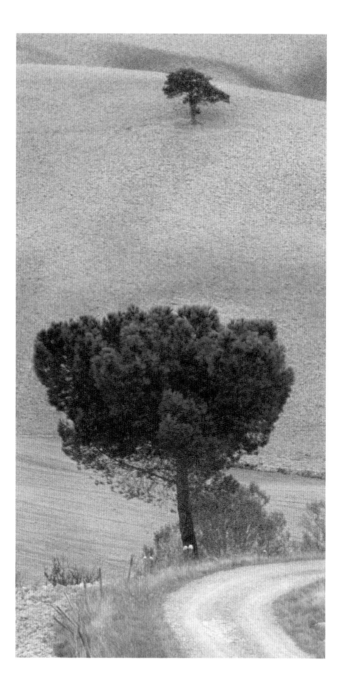

EXERCISE 25 ❖ SAT KRIYA

Sit on the heels in Rock Pose, arms straight above head. Fingers interlock in Venus Lock with Jupiter (index) fingers pointing straight up. Arms hug the ears (Fig. 25A1) with the elbows locked straight.

Venus Lock channels sexual energy and promotes glandular balance. To form the Venus Lock, place the palms facing each other. Interlace the fingers with the left little finger on the bottom. Men should put the left thumb tip just above the base of the thumb on the webbing between the thumb and index finger. The tip of the right thumb presses the fleshy mound at the base of the left thumb (Fig. 25A2). For women, the thumb positions and all the other fingers, are reversed (Fig. 25A3); the left thumb is on the outside and the fingers alternate so the right little finger is also on the outside. Then place the Jupiter fingers together making a steeple, and bring the arms up with index fingers pointing straight up (Fig. 25A4).

As you say "Sat" aloud, apply Mool Bhand by tensing the rectum and sex organs, pulling them up to the navel point as you pull the navel point into the spine. As you say "Naam" aloud, release the navel. Keep rectum and sex organ held. The breath will regulate itself. Be sure that you do it slowly enough to pull the locks completely, continuing this rhythm for 3 to 31 minutes. The sound means "truth is my identity."

To end, inhale, apply the full Mool Bhand, exhale and relax. This exercise will make every gland and organ in the body secrete, for it is the most powerful kriya known to man. This exercise may be done in a group, but not for the full 31 minutes. Practicing by yourself, you can practice for 3 to 31 minutes.

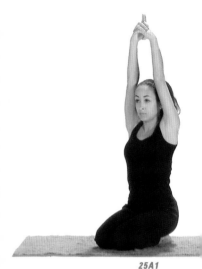

25A1

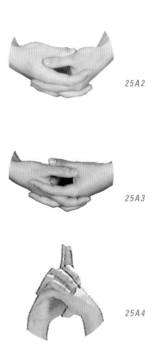

25A2

25A3

25A4

BENEFITS

Sat Kriya is one of the first exercises Yogi Bhajan taught his first students in the Western world over thirty years ago. It stimulates the navel point (adjusting all 72,000 major nerves in the body), massages all the internal organs, causes the entire endocrine gland system to secrete, and directly stimulates the kundalini energy stored at the base of the spine so that you can experience your unknown potential self.

Total Time: 3–31 minutes

CHAPTER TWENTYSIX
Find the Compass of Your Soul

Every once in a while, it is useful to check your bearings and discover whether your current direction in life is consistent with what you have to accomplish. Yogis have the perspective that every person has a purpose in life, a mission to fulfill. The Meditation on the Self (Meditation 26) can help you find the compass of your soul.

According to Yogi Bhajan, every person has two potential destinies: what our life would be like if we acted from our highest consciousness (the "projected destiny"), versus what our life would be like if we did not act that way (the destiny or fate).

Another way of saying this is that when you act in higher consciousness, you follow a path of *dharma* (righteous living); otherwise, you suffer the *karma* (consequences) of past actions.

MEDITATION 26 ❖ MEDITATION ON THE SELF

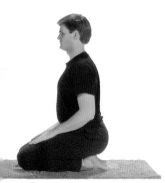

26A

1. Spine Flex. Sit on the heels with palms down on the thighs.

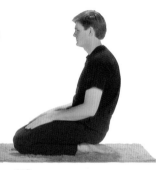

26B

Flex the spine forward and back rhythmically. Begin the Breath of Fire. The spine will move slower than the breath, keeping an even pace. Concentrate at the brow point. Continue for 3 minutes, then inhale, hold, and relax the breath.

2. Sat Kriya. Immediately bring the hands over the head, arms hugging the ears and the palms flat together. Begin Sat Kriya, rhythmically pulling the navel in as you say "Sat," relaxing it as you say "Naam." Continue for 3 minutes, then inhale, hold the breath and apply Mool Bhand. Exhale, hold the breath out and again apply Mool Bhand. Relax.

26C

3. Sit in Easy Pose. Place the palms on the knees and alternately lift the shoulders in a smooth, moderately paced rhythm. Do Breath of Fire for 3 minutes.

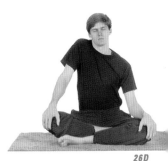

26D

4. Immediately sit in Easy Pose and meditate deeply. Feel the energy flow up along the spine. Let the light shine from your head to guide you in the path of truth. Meditate on your past. Meditate on your present. Who are you? Meditate on your future. What do you have to accomplish? You are created by the Creator to express Himself. Meditate deeply for 6 minutes, and repeat

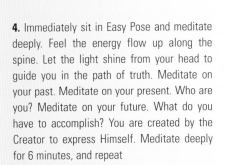

26E

26F

The mind is given to you to use in self-expansion. But you do not channel it or capture it. It runs wild on old thought patterns and habits. If you cannot have the mind when you need it, it is useless. The function of mind is not just to spew out random thoughts! It is to fashion etheric elements into forms of energy that manifest through the earthly elements. A projected imagination that is guided is a fundamental power and gift of mankind.

In this simple series, you raise the kundalini energy enough to purify and calm the mind. Then you direct the mind in meditation to become aware of your identity and how you have guided it. You use the mind for self-observation, not just fantasy.

BENEFITS

Besides being excellent training for the mind, this kriya helps improve poor digestion and channels overabundant sexual energy. In a few minutes, the mind can become focused. This is one of the beauties of Kundalini Yoga. Instead of dealing with thoughts only with other thoughts, it uses exercises that automatically bring the mind into a more meditative state. This saves years of meditation time. The body is your finite identity. The mind is a bridge to your infinite identity, which is even beyond the soul. But the mind alone has a difficult time since it lacks the clarity of identity given by the body. When you manipulate the body identity by exercises, then a clear message of guidance is given to the mind. It is not the mind that runs the body. It is actually you. The mind is another part of you. Using these two to communicate with and integrate your many parts is the science of kriya and a basis of Kundalini Yoga.

Total Time: 15–30 minutes

CHAPTER TWENTYSEVEN
Connecting With Your Totality

Sodarshan Chakra Kriya (Meditation 27) is not easy to do, but this book would not be complete without its inclusion because it is so powerful, effective, and comprehensive.

Yogi Bhajan has recommended this exercise as a key tool in transitioning yourself into the Aquarian Age during the critical cusp period (during the years 1991–2012) leading from the Piscean Age into the Aquarian Age.

You can begin with a few minutes' practice and gradually work your way up to practicing for longer durations at a session. The return on investment in elevating your consciousness is great, and warrants the effort. Try this meditation and see what it does for you.

MEDITATION 27 ❖ SODARSHAN CHAKRA KRIYA

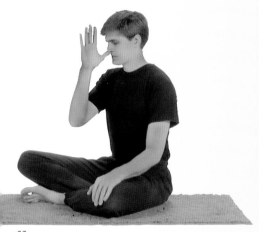

Sit in Easy Pose with a straight spine. Eyes are fixed at the tip of the nose or eyes are closed, as you prefer. Block off the right nostril with the right thumb. Inhale slowly and deeply through the left nostril. Hold the breath.

Mentally chant "Wah-hay Guroo" sixteen times, pumping the navel point three times with each repetition, once on "Wah," once on "Hay," and once on "Guroo"—for a total of forty-eight pumps.

27

Then unblock the right nostril. Place the right index finger (or the little finger can also be used) to block off the left nostril, and exhale slowly and deeply through the right nostril.

Continue for 31 to 62 minutes. Suggested length for this kriya is 31 minutes or 62 minutes a day.

To end the meditation: inhale, hold the breath 5 to 10 seconds, exhale. Then stretch and shake every part of your body for about 1 minute so that the energy may spread.

This is how Yogi Bhajan keeps track of the counting:

Blocking the right nostril with the right thumb, other fingers held straight up in the air, he holds the breath and counts to sixteen with his fingers, as follows.

One, two, three — *counted with the little finger of the right hand, moving it slightly three times.*

Four, five, six — *moving the ring finger three times.*

Seven, eight, nine — *moving the middle finger three times.*

Ten, eleven, twelve — *moving the index finger three times.*

Thirteen, fourteen, fifteen — *moving the thumb slightly for three beats.*

Sixteen — *bringing the index finger over to block off the left nostril as he releases the right thumb from the right nostril. Then he exhales through the right nostril.*

Time Constraints: *There is no time, no place, no space, and no condition attached to this mantra. Each garbage pit has its own time to clear. If you are going to clean your own garbage, you must estimate and clean it as fast as you can, or as slow as you want.* You *have to decide how much time you have to clean up your garbage pit.*

BENEFITS

This is the highest kriya in all of yoga. This meditation cuts through all darkness. It will give you a new start. It is the simplest kriya, but at the same time the hardest. It cuts through all barriers of the neurotic or psychotic inside-nature. When a person is in a very bad state, techniques imposed from the outside will not work. The pressure has to be stimulated from within.

Tragedy of life is when the subconscious releases garbage into the conscious mind. This kriya invokes the kundalini to give you the necessary vitality and intuition to combat the negative effects of the subconscious mind.

Total Time: 31–62 minutes

Yogi Bhajan says of this meditation: If you can do this meditation for 62 minutes to start with and develop to the point that you can do it 2½ hours a day, it will give you the following: *Nao niddhi, athara siddhi.* **Nine precious virtues and eighteen occult powers. And in those twenty-seven total virtues of the world**

lies the entire universe. So start with 31 minutes, then after a while (weeks or months) do it for 40 minutes, then for 62 minutes. Take time to graduate in it.

When practiced 2½ hours every day, it makes out of you a perfect superman. It purifies, it takes care of the human life, and brings together all twenty-seven facets of life and makes a human perfect, saintly, successful, and qualified. This meditation also gives one the pranic power. This kriya never fails. It can give one all the inner happiness, and bring one to a state of ecstasy in life.

CHAPTER TWENTY-EIGHT
Inspiration

For over twenty-five years, I have used the Five Sutras of the Aquarian Age as a kind of Swiss Army knife for life. It is an essential tool kit for dealing with the stresses of everyday life. It features a hammer, a knife, a screwdriver, a wrench, and a pair of pliers for all situations in your life.

About thirty years ago, during the time between college and beginning to work in the corporate arena, I lived for a time atop a hill in the foothills of the California Sierras in a small A-frame cabin without electricity or running water—an environment suitable for the spiritual quest to discover myself. The roof of the cabin had rain troughs that collected rainwater and funneled it into a circular water tank. I read books by kerosene lantern, including *The Life of Milarepa, Tibet's Greatest Yogi.* I learned self-reliance. I also learned that when the water in the water tank tastes funny, it is time to make sure a mouse has not fallen into it. I learned that the pocketknife is an invaluable tool to a mountain man. By great good fortune some visiting friends had begun practicing yoga and I took a Kundalini Yoga class. I immediately knew this was the technology I had been seeking for my entire life and I resolved to teach it and share it with the world.

After practicing yoga every day for several months, I came down off my mountain top in May 1972 to take a teacher training course in

Kundalini Yoga. I had heard there was an annual event in June called Summer Solstice where yogis gathered and Yogi Bhajan taught, so I decided to go. That year it took place along the northern California coast near Mendocino. I went first to the San Francisco Bay Area, to a 3HO *ashram* (yoga center) in San Raphael where I met Yogi Bhajan for the first time. I asked his permission to attend Summer Solstice for free since I did not have the hundred dollars it cost to attend. "We are not beggars; you can earn it," he said. He also told me, "Be great." Those were probably the most important words anybody ever said to me.

The situation was a challenge because I only had thirty-five dollars and it was more money than I had had in a long time. But I had a month to earn the money, so I joined some folks who were picking organic oranges in southern California and selling them in the Bay Area. Then their truck broke down; I had to kick in all my savings to help get it fixed. Two weeks later, we delivered a truckload of oranges to a Bay Area health food store. Afterwards I was meditating at a house in Marin when it occurred to me that Summer Solstice attendees might like to eat organic oranges. I called up the cook, Jagdish Singh, and he invited us over immediately to provide a sample. He ordered two truckloads of organic oranges for Summer Solstice, and in partial payment, I got to attend.

We picked oranges for the next two weeks, and arrived at the camp on the first day. We formed a bucket brigade from the truck, up the hill and all the way to the kitchen, and unloaded bag after bag of oranges. There were hundreds of young people like myself, yogis working around the camp, singing, dancing, chanting, lots of children, majestic trees in full summer green, swirling wind, happy laughter . . . I was home.

It wasn't until a few years after I began practicing Kundalini Yoga that I discovered Yogi Bhajan had shared this teaching:

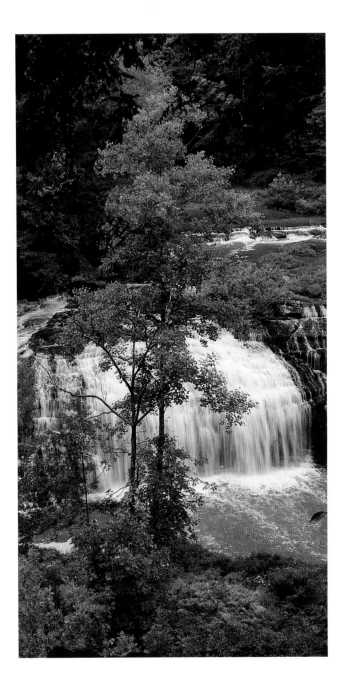

The Five Sutras of the Aquarian Age

1. **Recognize that the other person is you.**

2. **There is a way through every block.**

3. **When the time is on you, start, and the pressure will be off.**

4. **Understand through compassion or you will misunderstand the times.**

5. **Vibrate the Cosmos, Cosmos shall clear the path.**

— **Yogi Bhajan**

If you have ever heard the song "Aquarius" from the musical *Hair*, then you know that the Age of Aquarius (which gets into full swing by the year 2012 according to Yogi Bhajan — we are in the cusp period now that began in 1991) is an epoch of world peace, universal brotherhood, and love.

Humanity has a long way to go and many changes to go through before we get to that state of collective empathy and acceptance. But the Five Sutras of the Aquarian Age can help you reach that state. (A *sutra* is like a gem of thought, a diamond idea that can cut through anything.)

Just like that indispensable pocketknife, pick out the tool you need at any particular moment, and apply it.

My personal favorite sutra is number two, "There is a way through every block." It is a surefire antidote to depression, because it always gives you hope. A situation may seem hopeless, but this sutra explains that you just need to figure out how to work through the problem, which is much less stressful than the feeling that there is no way out.

Number three, "When the time is on you, start, and the pressure will be off," is great for reducing your stress. If you are feeling stressed out about some situation, it usually is because you have not started working on that situation. As soon as you start, you are in the flow of it, and the stress goes away.

Many people ask about number five: What is "Vibrate the Cosmos"? It means sounding a mantra such as "Sat Naam" or any of the other mantras described in this book, which are a key but small subset of the many mantras in Kundalini Yoga that can awaken you to the Infinite within you.

I have the Five Sutras printed on the back of my business cards. When I travel and get assistance from someone I may never meet again, handing out this card makes a great way to thank someone when you only have a few moments.

I hope you derive as much soul satisfaction from applying these tools to your life as I have. Please let me know how things turn out when you apply the tools provided in this book to your life.

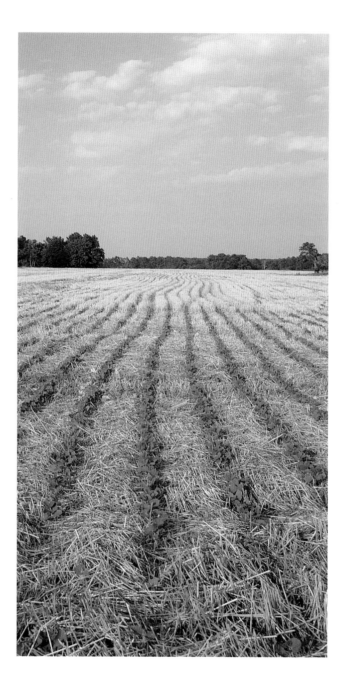

APPENDICES

Mudras

Modern medical science has mapped out regions of the brain surface that correlate to the physical body and discovered that more neurons are dedicated to sensory input from, and control of, the face and hands than any other parts of the body. Sight, hearing, smell, and taste are all localized in the face. Face to face communication among humans takes place through speech, facial expression, and hand/body gestures, so the ability to control face and hands, and to recognize what is being communicated through these instruments, has been critical to our survival and success as social animals for millions of years.

The hands are energy maps of our consciousness. Yogis long ago mapped out the hand areas and their different neural reflexes in the brain. Each area of the hands correlates to a corresponding area of the brain on a particular brain hemisphere, and each area also represents different emotions or behaviors. Yogis recognized that by curling, crossing, stretching, and touching the fingers and hands in various ways, we can effectively communicate with our own body and mind. In the same way that telephone switchboard operators in the early twentieth century made connections between different callers by plugging cables into various circuits, specific hand postures (mudras) can communicate clear messages to the body/mind energy system. Each of the basic mudras listed below is used in meditation to enhance specific energy patterns in the brain.

GYAN MUDRA

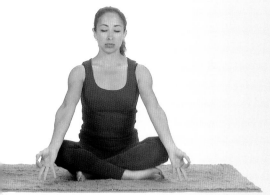

Mudra 1

To form passive Gyan Mudra, put the tip of the thumb together with the tip of the index finger (Fig. Mudra 1). This stimulates your knowledge and ability. The energy of the index finger is often symbolized by Jupiter, the planet representing expansion. This mudra is the one most commonly used. It gives you receptivity and calmness.

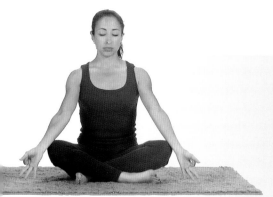

Mudra 2

In the practice of powerful pranayams or exercises, the active form of Gyan Mudra is often used. In this case, you bend the index finger under the thumb so the fingernail is on the second joint of the thumb (Fig. Mudra 2).

SHUNI MUDRA

To form Shuni Mudra, place the tip of the middle finger on the tip of the thumb (Fig. Mudra 3). This mudra is said to give patience and discernment. The middle finger is often symbolized by the planet Saturn. Saturn represents the task master, the law of karma, the taking of responsibility, and the courage to hold to duty.

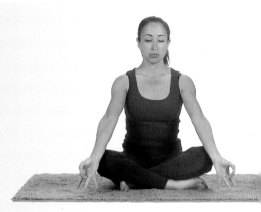

Mudra 3

SURYA MUDRA

Surya Mudra (also called Ravi Mudra) is formed by placing the tip of the ring finger on the tip of the thumb (Fig. Mudra 4). Practicing it gives revitalizing energy, nervous strength, and good health. The quality of the ring finger is symbolized by the sun or Uranus. The sun represents energy, health, and sexuality. Uranus stands for nerve strength, intuition, and change.

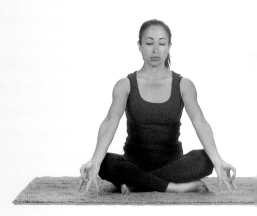

Mudra 4

BUDDHI MUDRA

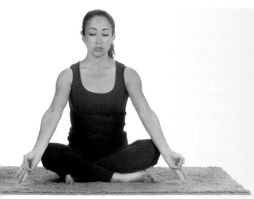

To form Buddhi Mudra, place the tip of the little finger on the tip of the thumb (Fig. Mudra 5). Practicing this opens the capacity to communicate clearly and intuitively. It also stimulates psychic development. The little finger is symbolized by Mercury for quickness and the mental powers of communication.

Mudra 5

VENUS LOCK

This mudra is used frequently in exercises. It derives the name because it connects the positive and negative sides of the Venus mound on each hand to the thumbs. The thumbs represent the ego. The Venus mound is the fleshy area at the base of the thumb. It is symbolized by the planet Venus, which is associated with the energy of sensuality and sexuality. The mudra channels the sexual energy and promotes glandular balance. It also brings the ability to focus or concentrate easily if you rest it in your lap while in a meditative posture. To form the mudra, place the palms facing each other. Interlace the fingers alternately with the left little finger on the bottom. Put the left thumb tip just above the base of the right thumb on the webbing between the thumb and index finger. The tip of the right thumb presses the fleshy mound at the base of the left thumb (Fig. Mudra 6A). Thumb positions and all the other fingers are reversed for women (Fig. Mudra 6B); the left thumb is on the outside and the fingers alternate so the right little finger is also on the outside.

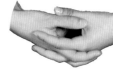

Mudra 6A

Mudra 6B

PRAYER MUDRA

For this, the palms of the hands are flat together (Fig. Mudra 7). The positive side of the body (right, or male) and negative (left, or female) are neutralized. This is always used when initially centering yourself by Tuning In in preparation for doing a kriya.

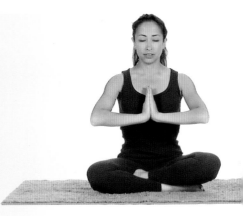

Mudra 7

HANDS IN LAP

Another common mudra for meditation is formed by resting the left palm face-up in the lap with the right hand palm up on top of it (Fig. Mudra 8). Put the thumb tips together. The hand positions are usually reversed for a woman.

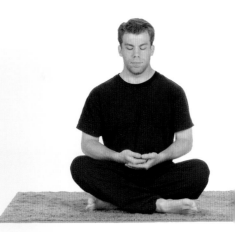

Mudra 8

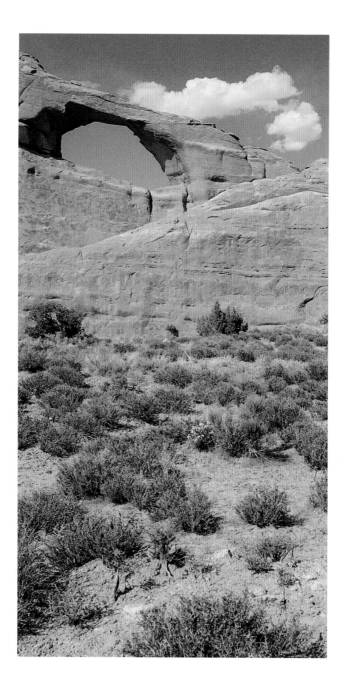

Mantras

Chanting a mantra is a method of tuning your mind to a particular vibratory frequency, in much the same way that you can tune a television in to a particular channel to receive information on that channel.

Whatever you focus your mind on will eventually manifest. If you focus a great deal of mental energy on "money, money, money," then you may eventually be surrounded by money. But if you don't also focus on developing the capacity to handle the responsibility of all this money, you may wind up even more miserable than before.

So the best strategy is to focus the mind on the highest and most uplifting frequencies possible. Therefore, yogic mantras consist of specific sounds, typically words derived from the Sanskrit language or its derivatives, designed to align your being with the fundamental frequencies of the universe.

Mantra works because of the yogic principle: *japa* (repetition of a mantra) creates *tapa* (psychic heat). The mental friction of repeating a mantra is considered to gradually burn up negative thought patterns and desires in the mind.

All the mantras in Kundalini Yoga are designed to tune the mind into the Infinite that pervades the creation. The vibratory frequency— the sound—that is generated when you chant, either aloud or silently, is called the *Naad* or "sound current" by the yogis. The combination of Naad with various yoga postures, breathing patterns, and movement is a very powerful way to influence the psyche and elevate consciousness.

Chanting aloud is effective because it stimulates the nervous system and the brain. There are eighty-four meridians (nerve endings) in the upper palate of the mouth that lead directly into the brain, and they are stimulated by the movement of the tongue against the upper palate when you chant or speak. Because chanting resonates sound in the skull and brain, and this sound reenters the brain through the ears, various patterns of neurons in the brain are triggered by these sounds. Therefore, whatever you say directly affects your consciousness. When you chant the scientific sounds of a mantra, which is designed to affect your nervous system so that the sounds do to you what they mean, the effect can be very elevating to your consciousness.

Mantras may be chanted mentally while doing yoga, while sitting in meditation, or at any time in coordination with your breath throughout the day, to center, calm, energize and elevate yourself. Here are the mantras used in this book:

ONG NAMO GUROO DAYV NAMO

"Creator, I bow, Wisdom present everywhere, I bow." Always use this mantra to tune in to the wisdom within you before practicing yoga.

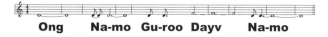

Ong   **Na-mo Gu-roo Dayv**   **Na-mo**

SAT NAAM

"Truth is my identity." Use this mantra with every breath throughout your yoga practice unless otherwise specified. This *beej* (seed) mantra is the most commonly used mantra in Kundalini Yoga. When chanting Long Sat Naam on a full breath, the duration of the word "Sat" is extended in duration, as follows:

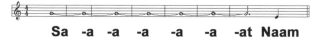

Sa -a -a -a   -a   -a -at Naam

SAA TAA NAA MAA

"Creation Life Death Rebirth." These are the five primal sounds (four consonants and a vowel) that control the inner universe. In this mantra, the molecular energy of truth (*Sat Naam*) is broken down into its component sounds, unleashing energy to cleanse the subconscious mind.

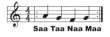

Saa Taa Naa Maa

HAR HARAY HAREE, WAH-HAY GUROO

This mantra stimulates *Har* (creativity) into action. *Wah-hay Guroo* means "Infinite Wisdom."

GOBIND

"Sustainer" is an attribute of Infinity.

GUROO GUROO WAH-HAY GUROO, GUROO RAAM DAAS GUROO

"Wise, wise is the one who serves Infinity." This meditation brings protection, relaxation, self-healing, and emotional relief.

Gu-roo Gu-roo Wah-hay Gu-roo, Gu-roo Raam Daas Gu-roo

Repeat once

Gu-roo Gu-roo Wah-hay Gu-roo, Gu-roo Raam Daas Gu-roo

Repeat line 1 once

WAH-HAY GUROO

Wah-hay means "inexpressible, beyond words." *Guroo* is the wisdom of the universe. This is a *beej* (seed) mantra and the second most commonly used mantra in Kundalini Yoga.

HARING

"Creator." This mantra expresses the creativity of the universe in action.

HAREE HAR, HAREE HAR, HAREE HAR, HAREE HAR, HAREE HAR, HAREE HAR, HAREE HAR, HAREE HAR

Haree means "creative action." *Har* means "creativity." This mantra contrasts, respectively, the kinetic and potential energy of creativity so that you can distinguish between them. Meditating on this mantra leads to a deeper understanding of the source of creativity and how it manifests in the universe.

RAA RAA RAA RAA, MAA MAA MAA MAA, SAA SAA SAA SAT, HAREE HAR HAREE HAR

Raa evokes the "father" energy within you. *Maa* evokes the "mother" energy within you. *Saa* means "creation" and *Sat* means "truth." *Haree Har* is creativity in motion. Together these sounds stimulate within you an appreciation for the cosmic creativity of the union of male and female polarities in the universe.

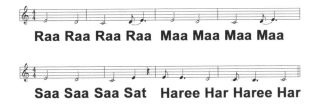

Raa Raa Raa Raa Maa Maa Maa Maa

Saa Saa Saa Sat Haree Har Haree Har

HA REE, HA REE, HA REE, HA REE, HA REE, HA REE, HAR

In this mantra, the molecular energy of creativity (Haree) is broken down into its component sounds, unleashing great creative potential. This sound evokes healing within you, and opens you up to new possibilities.

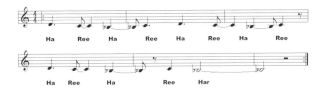

Ha Ree Ha Ree Ha Ree Ha Ree

Ha Ree Ha Ree Har

SAT NARAYAN WAH-HAY GUROO, HAREE NARAYAN SAT NAAM, SAT NARAYAN WAH-HAY GUROO, HAREE NARAYAN SAT NAAM

Sat Narayan means "true sustainer." *Haree Narayan* means "creative sustenance." This mantra develops clarity of mind.

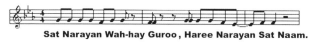

Sat Narayan Wah-hay Guroo , Haree Narayan Sat Naam.

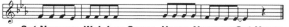

Sat Narayan Wah-hay Guroo, Haree Narayan Sat Naam.

Glossary of Terms

Term	Definition
Aquarian Age	According to astrology, the Aquarian Age is a two-thousand-year period from year 2000 to 3999 during which world peace and universal brotherhood shall prevail.
Asana	One of a series of body postures practiced during yoga exercise.
Aura	The human electromagnetic field that surrounds the physical body.
Autonomic Nervous System	A part of the body's nervous system that governs involuntary activities such as digestion and heartbeat, consisting of the parasympathetic and sympathetic nervous systems.
Breath of Fire	One of the most effective breathing exercises for healing the body. It strengthens the nervous system, purifies the blood and stimulates the endocrine gland system.
Breath Rate	Breath is the gift of life. By controlling the breath rate, the yoga practitioner alters his/her state of mind.
Brow Point	Some meditations involve mental concentration at a point on the forehead slightly above where the root of the nose meets the eyebrows, known as the brow point or third eye point.
Charisma	A special magnetic charm or appeal of a person. The yogic perspective is that charisma is the effect of a person's strong electromagnetic field or aura.

Term	Definition
Cold Depression	Depression occurs when the human body cannot keep up with the needs of the time and circumstances. The chaos of information in the computer age will make it difficult for people to cope with their day-to-day lives.
Dharma	Righteous living wherein one follows a way of life that adheres to spiritual principles such as truthfulness, earning an honest living, and sharing with others.
Diaphragm Lock	A body posture that lifts the diaphragm up high into the thorax, usually applied with the breath held out. This regulates the flow of energy around the heart.
Easy Pose	A comfortable cross-legged sitting posture.
Golden Chain	Psychic connection between you and your yoga teacher, to his teacher, and so on unto Infinity.
Gyan Mudra	A specific hand posture designed to put your ego under the direction of your wisdom. There are sixteen variants of this mudra.
Jalandhara Bhand	See Neck Lock
Karma	The consequences of previous actions, wherein you reap what you sow. Yogis consider that Dharmic living is an antidote to negative karmas from previous lifetimes.

Term	Definition
Kirtan Kriya	A musical meditation for cleansing the subconscious mind.
Kriya	A complete set of yoga exercises sequenced to achieve a specific result.
Kundalini	The nerve of the soul, stored at the base of the spine. When its energy is awakened, which is the goal of yoga, it uncoils up the spine to the top of the head and the person experiences higher consciousness.
Kundalini Yoga	A comprehensive and effective form of yoga that offers an immediate and direct effect in a short amount of time.
Left Nostril Breathing	Left nostril breathing lowers the body temperature, lowers the blood pressure, and soothes the emotions.
Mantra	Specific words chanted aloud or silently to elevate one's state of mind. The sounds of a mantra are coded to stimulate some of the eighty-four nerve endings in the mouth and upper palate to affect the brain and raise consciousness.
Mastery	Mastery of a meditation means that the state of mind you are in during the meditation becomes immediately accessible to you at other times, just by thinking about it.
Meditation	A form of sustained concentration during which one's flow of thoughts becomes calmer and more focused.

Term	Definition
Mool Bhand	A body posture that contracts the muscles of the rectum, sex organ, and navel point to move energy up the spine; also known as Root Lock.
Mudra	A specific hand posture designed to affect energy flow in the brain during meditation.
Naad	The vibratory frequency created by chanting mantras.
Nabhi Kriya	A navel-strengthening exercise set.
Navel Point	The belly button and the nerve complex behind it.
Neck Lock	A body posture that makes the neck straight in line with the rest of the spine. Neck lock is applied by pulling the chin in toward the Adam's apple, thus regulating the flow of energy and blood into the brain.
Panj Shabd Mantra	The mantra *Saa Taa Naa Maa* which cleanses the subconscious mind.
Parasympathetic Nervous System	A part of the autonomic nervous system governing involuntary activities that tends to induce glandular secretion, increase the contraction of smooth muscle tissue, and cause the dilatation of blood vessels.
Pineal Gland	Yogis consider this endocrine gland within the brain to be the source of higher consciousness when it secretes.

Term	Definition
Pituitary Gland	The master endocrine gland that regulates all the other endocrine glands. Yogis consider this endocrine gland within the brain to be the source of intuition when it secretes. The projection of the pituitary energy is focused at the brow point, also known as the third eye point in mystical traditions around the world.
Prana	Energy of the life force that comes in the breath. Yoga practitioners practice breathing exercises to increase the amount of prana in the body for improved health and healing.
Pranam Mudra	A body posture of greeting someone with open arms.
Pranayam	A breathing exercise practiced in a particular pattern to adjust the level of prana in the body.
Right Nostril Breathing	Right nostril breathing raises the body temperature, raises the blood pressure, and charges you up with physical energy.
Root Lock	See Mool Bhand
Sat Kriya	A powerful exercise for raising the kundalini energy.
Sat Naam	Most commonly used mantra in Kundalini Yoga. Loosely translated, it means "truth."
Shabd	Sound
Sitali Pranayam	A cooling and healing breath useful in ridding the body of disease.

Term	Definition
Stress	Stress is the body's primitive reaction to challenging environments and circumstances. Stress can eat up your life, ruin your career and your health, and (through the release of cortisol in your bloodstream), even kills brain cells.
Sutra	A string of thoughts like a necklace constituting a series of powerful ideas.
Sympathetic Nervous System	A part of the autonomic nervous system governing involuntary activities that tends to reduce glandular secretion, decrease the contraction of smooth muscle tissue, and cause the contraction of blood vessels.
Tattvas	The five alchemical elements (fire, air, water, earth, and ether) are categories of quality that are based in the energetic flow of your life force. If all the elements are strong, in balance, and are located in their proper areas of the body, then you can resist stress, trauma and illness.
Third Eye Point	Focusing the eyes at the third eye point stimulates the pituitary gland and causes it to secrete. See Brow Point, Pituitary Gland.

Term	Definition
Venus Lock	A hand position (mudra) often used to balance energy in the body. This mudra derives its name from the connection the thumbs make between the positive and negative sides of the Venus mound on each hand. The mudra channels the sexual energy and promotes glandular balance. This mudra brings the ability to focus or concentrate when the hands are rested in the lap while sitting in a meditative posture such as Easy Pose.
Wah-hay Guroo	Mantra meaning "inexpressible wisdom."
Yoga	Yoga is a science of the mind, an ancient system of exercise that includes thousands of physical and mental exercises designed to strengthen and balance the body, rejuvenate the nervous system, and concentrate the mind. Yoga integrates body and mind so that you can experience your essence: inner peace. The goal of yoga is to develop self-mastery, to be consciously conscious so that your actions are wholehearted and balanced, to unite your sense of a limited and finite personal self with your capacity as part of the unlimited spirit and consciousness.
Yogi	Someone who practices yoga. Used as a person's title, Yogi refers to someone who has mastered yoga.

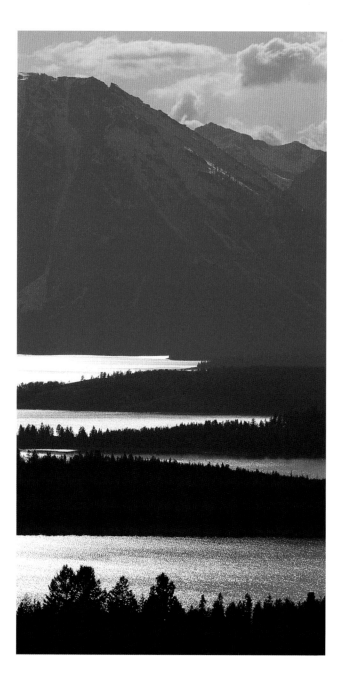

Resources

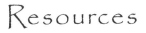

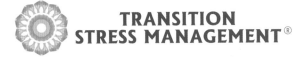

TRANSITION STRESS MANAGEMENT®

Transition Stress Management (TSM) provides business innovation consulting and stress management services through its global services delivery network directly to corporate clients at their facilities around the world. For further information, check the website: www.transitionstressmanage.com, or send an email message to YogaSecrets@transitionstressmanage.com.

BALANCED GROUP THINKING®

Transition Stress Management provides Balanced Group Thinking services, a transformational group experience custom-designed to move management and operational teams to new perspectives and unleash creativity. Balanced Group Thinking is a powerful teambuilding methodology that combines yoga meditation and storyboarding in a unique patent-pending process for world-class innovation. Applications include strategic planning, problem solving, project management, and business process re-engineering, conflict resolution, and more. For further information, check the website: www.balancedgroupthinking.com.

KUNDALINI YOGA

Kundalini Yoga classes are offered to the general public through certified Kundalini Yoga teachers around the world, many of whom are members of the International Kundalini Yoga Teachers Association. Check the following websites for further information:

- International Kundalini Yoga Teachers Association: www.kundaliniyoga.com to locate a Kundalini Yoga teacher or training center nearest you.

- 3HO Foundation: www.3ho.org for more information about Kundalini Yoga and 3HO courses and events around the world.

- Yogi Bhajan: www.yogibhajan.com for more information about the teachings of Yogi Bhajan.

BREATHWALK

Breathwalk is the science of combining specific patterns of breathing synchronized with your walking steps and enhanced with the art of directed meditative attention. Breathwalk is a simple, natural, and effective technique for physical and mental fitness, enhanced mood, mental clarity, and physical energy. For further information, check the website: www.breathwalk.com.

ANCIENT HEALING WAYS

An excellent source for books, music, and videos, including Yogi Bhajan lectures on audiotape and videotape. Also available: Yogi Tea products, yogic formulas, and lifestyle products associated with Kundalini Yoga including Peace Cereals. Check the website: www.a-healing.com for online purchases, or call 800-359-2940. Many of the music and books referenced in this book are available there.

GRD CENTER FOR MEDICINE AND HUMANOLOGY

This charitable research center provides yoga therapy and Sat Nam Rasayan healing technology for health recovery of persons living with chronic or life-threatening illness. For further information, check the website: www.grdcenter.org, or call 800-326-1322.

AMAR INFINITY FOUNDATION

Amar Infinity Foundation seeks, receives, and expends philanthropic funds for nonprofit organizations such as 3HO Foundation, Kundalini Research Institute, Sikh Dharma, Sikh Dharma Education International and their affiliated programs, insuring their longevity by providing funding to meet short- and long-term goals. You can support these efforts and ensure their legacy through a variety of gifting and estate planning programs. For further information, check the website: www.amarinfinity.org.

LIVSKRAFT MANAGEMENT

Livskraft Management is an affiliate of the Transition Stress Management global service delivery network, providing Kundalini Yoga classes to major corporations in Sweden. For further information, check the website: www.lkm-imy.com.

THE ALZHEIMER'S PREVENTION FOUNDATION

This foundation has a mission in the prevention and reversal of memory loss. For further information, check the website: www.brain-longevity.com.

THE CLEANSE

The Cleanse is a service that offers a synergistic combination of a specific diet, Chinese herbs, extra supplements, Kundalini Yoga, and meditation to purify body, mind, and spirit. The Cleanse uses detoxifying and strengthening methods to re-establish your body's integrity at a cellular level, and works to give you the tools to restore, and then maintain, a state of optimal health, vitality, and aliveness. For further information, check the website: www.thecleanse.com, or call 800-563-3327.

WOMANHEART

Healing, Kundalini Yoga, and women's retreats around the country. Check the website: www.womanheart.com.

SPIRIT VOYAGE

Beautiful meditation music. The sounds of the ancient Eastern cultures merged with the styles and techniques of the modern West. For further information, check the website: www.spiritvoyage.com, or call 888-735-4800.

SACRED GEMS

A source for malas (meditation beads) and healing gemstones. Check the website: www.sacredgems.com

GREAT SMOKIES DIAGNOSTIC LABORATORY

This testing service offers some allergen tests you can obtain through your physician. Check the website: www.gsdl.com, or call 800-522-4762.

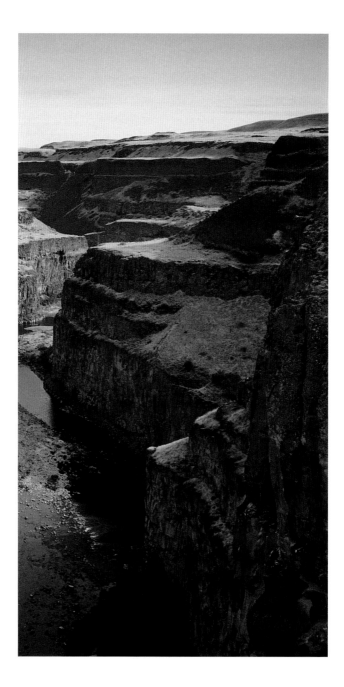

Recommended Reading

Khalsa, Nirvair Singh. *Heal Your Back Now!* Anchorage, 1998.

Khalsa, Shakta Kaur. *Kundalini Yoga.* Dorling Kindersley, New York, 2001.

Khalsa, Shakti Parwha Kaur. *Kundalini Yoga, The Flow of Eternal Power.* Perigee Books, New York, 1999.

Yogi Bhajan. *Golden Temple Vegetarian Cookbook.* South Asia Books, 1999.

Yogi Bhajan and Gurucharan Singh Khalsa, *Breathwalk.* Broadway Books, New York, 2000.

———— *The Mind, Its Projections and Multiple Facets.* Kundalini Research Institute, New Mexico, 1998.

About Yogi Bhajan

Yogi Bhajan is a Master of Kundalini Yoga and a dedicated and inspired teacher. In 1969, he left a successful twenty-year career in service to the government of India in order to bring to America the yogic and meditative technology in which he had been extensively trained from an early age. He founded the 3HO Foundation, the "Healthy, Happy, Holy Organization," a nonprofit organization dedicated to the advancement of the individual and the upliftment of humanity through education, science, and religion. 3HO teaches a unique blend of the proven ancient technologies of the East and the modern scientific innovations of the West so that all who wish may live healthily, happily and "wholly" in all aspects of life. Yogi Bhajan has served as the Director of Spiritual Education for 3HO since its inception.

3HO Foundation is a Non-Governmental Organization (NGO) in Consultative Status with the Economic and Social Council of the United Nations. Today, 3HO Foundation is a worldwide association of people with over 300 teaching centers in 35 countries. Over 200 books and videos in many different languages have been written on Kundalini Yoga as taught by Yogi Bhajan.

In 1973, Yogi Bhajan founded 3HO SuperHealth, a successful addiction treatment program, blending the proven ancient wisdom of the East with the modern technology of the West. SuperHealth has been accredited by the prestigious Joint Commission on Accreditation of Healthcare Organizations and received its highest commendation. In 1978 it distinguished itself as being in the top 10 percent of all addiction treatment programs throughout the United States. In 1989, Yogi Bhajan met with Soviet President Mikhail Gorbachev, and established several addiction treatment programs in Russia based on the 3HO SuperHealth model.

As a world leader and a champion of world peace, Yogi Bhajan has been a strong promoter of inter-religious dialogue. He has championed human values, world peace, interfaith unity, and goodwill. He is a member of the World Parliament of Religions, and has been the Co-President of the Human Unity Conference, which has been held in India, Brazil, Canada, England, Mexico, and the United States. In 1990, he spoke at the Global Forum on the Environment in Moscow as an ambassador for the Sikhs. He has met with religious leaders around the world, and was a featured speaker at the United Nations Millennium Peace Summit held in August 2000.

Yogi Bhajan established the annual International Peace Prayer Day in June 1980. This day of prayer for world peace draws many prominent national and international leaders in the realms of religion, politics, and humanity. His ministry has worked side by side with religious leaders such as the Dalai Lama, the Archbishop of Canterbury, and prominent Hindu and Muslim leaders.

Yogi Bhajan is the Chief Management Advisor for fourteen corporations worldwide, active in diverse industries including health food manufacturing, computers, and security services. These companies have brought economic development to every community in which they participate.

Yogi Bhajan lectures and teaches throughout the world to audiences ranging from spiritual seekers to corporate executives to government dignitaries. He has written more than thirty books on topics including psychology, healing, and spirituality. He has taught and written extensively in the fields of natural health, utilizing herbal, ayurvedic, homeopathic, and yogic healing practices and formulas.

About the Author

Darshan Singh Khalsa is the founder and president of Transition Stress Management, Inc., an Arizona corporation founded in 1999 to provide

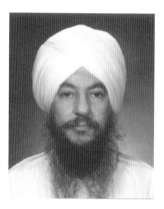

business innovation consulting and stress management services to meet the requirements of global corporations. Previously, Darshan provided management leadership in a fast-paced corporate environment for more than twenty years as one of the first employees of a Fortune 500 computer company.

For nearly a decade, he has provided consulting services such as strategic planning, team building and problem solving, project management, business process re-engineering, and Internet electronic commerce development for some of the world's largest corporations, including Carlson Companies, Citibank, Halliburton, Hewlett Packard, IBM, Kodak, MicroAge, Phillips Petroleum, PricewaterhouseCoopers, Southwestern Bell, and Wells Fargo Bank. He now provides business innovation services to organizations of all sizes.

Darshan is an internationally certified Kundalini Yoga and meditation teacher with thirty years' teaching experience under the direction of Yogi Bhajan, Master of Kundalini Yoga. He is a registered professional member of the International Kundalini Yoga Teachers Association, the International Yoga Association, and the Yoga Alliance, and is a master storyboarder mentored by Jim Norman of the Creative Planning Center of Phoenix, Arizona. He received the Storyboarder of the Year Award in 2001. He is also a member of the Society for Human Resource Management.

Darshan, author of several books on Kundalini Yoga, developed the Transition Stress Management corporate courseware comprising two years of sequenced Kundalini Yoga classes to optimize participants' health, nerve stamina, emotional well-being, and expanded consciousness.

Darshan is a Sikh, and a member of the International Khalsa Council of Sikh Dharma Western Hemisphere. Among other career highlights, in the mid–1970s he wrote screenplays for an independent Hollywood producer, and in the mid–1960s worked on the NASA Apollo Project as a computer programmer to help put man on the moon. He has lived in Phoenix, Arizona since 1972, and has a wife and one adult son.

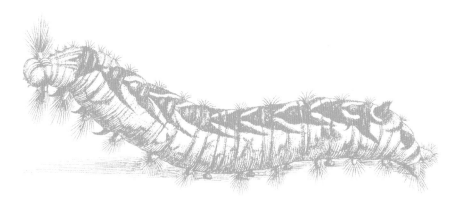

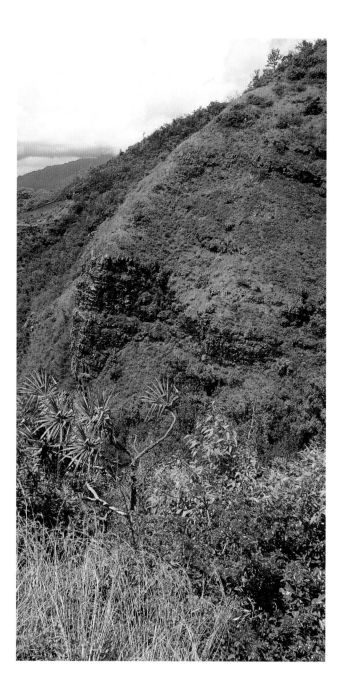

Endnotes

1. Abraham H. Maslow, *Motivation and Personality* (New York: Harper & Row, 1954).

2. Yogi Bhajan, 3HO Transcripts, unpublished lecture (November 2, 1993).

3. Yogi Bhajan and Gurucharan Singh Khalsa, monograph: "Shabd Guru: Basis, Usage and Impact of the Quantum Technology of the Shabd Guru" (April 1995), 5.

4. World Health Organization, *Fact Sheet N130* (August 1996), 1. "In the United States alone, depression costs some US $44 billion annually, which is about the same as the costs resulting from heart disease. It represents some 30 percent of the total estimated annual cost of US $148 billion for all mental illness."

5. World Health Organization/Harvard University, study: "The Global Burden of Disease: A Comprehensive Assessment of Mortality and Disability from Diseases, Injuries, and Risk Factors in 1990 and Projected to 2020" (1998), 1. "The next two decades will see dramatic changes in the health needs of the world's populations. In the developing regions where four-fifths of the planet's people live, non-communicable diseases such as depression and heart disease are fast replacing the traditional enemies, such as infectious diseases and malnutrition, as the leading causes of disability and premature death. By the year 2020, noncommunicable diseases are expected to account for seven out of every ten deaths in the developing regions, compared with less than half today."

6. Yogi Bhajan, "The Blue Gap" (lecture of April 12, 1973, Los Angeles, California) as quoted in *Beads of Truth* magazine (Los Angeles, California: 3HO Foundation, June 1973), 25.

7. John Naisbitt, "From Forced Technology to High Tech/High Touch," *MegaTrends* (New York: Warner Books, 1984), 35.

8. Yogi Bhajan, "The Nature and Need for a Spiritual Teacher," (lecture, February 14, 1972) as quoted in *The Possible Human* (IKYTA training manual by Yogi Bhajan and Gurucharan Singh Khalsa, "The Golden Link" chapter), 5-6.

Index

for Effective Communication,
135, 137–38
to Eliminate Stress, 38
to Feel and See Your Energy
Body, 131, 134
the Guru Mantra, 77, 80
for Hairtrigger Efficiency, 73, 75–76
to Heal the Physical, Mental, and
Spiritual bodies, 58–60
Kirtan Kriya, 149, 152–53, 155–56
Pranam Mudra, 65, 68–69
to Quell an Agitated Mind, 34
to Rejuvenate the Nervous
System, 53–56
to Relax and Rejoice, 105, 107–8
Sat Kriya, 157, 159–60, 162
Sat Narayan, 145, 147
on the Self, 161, 162–64
Shabd Kriya, 42–43
Smiling Buddha Kriya, 110–11
Sodarshan Chakra Kriya, 165–68
for Subconscious Temperamental
Anger, 85, 88
for Subconscious Temperamental
Fear, 70
Survasod, 139, 143–44
Tattva Balance Beyond Stress
and Quality, 129–30
for Transformation, 89, 91, 92–93, 95

menses, 17

mental illness, 126, 139

Mool Bhand, 13, 17, 114, 121, 159,
162

N

Nabhi Kriya, 118–22

Napoleon, 41

naval point, 13, 113, 117, 122, 160

Neck Lock, 10–11, 71

nervous system, 30, 46, 49, 50, 55,
59, 67, 75, 85, 113, 114, 117, 131

O

onions, 63

P

pancreas, 6

Panj Shabd. *See* mantras

parasympathetic system, 130

parathyroid, 6, 11

patience, 43, 85

Perfect Pose. *See* Rock Pose

phobias and fears, 65, 69, 126

pinial gland, 6, 11, 95, 126, 156

Piscean Age, 165

Pittar Kriya. *See* meditations

pituitary gland, 6, 11, 69, 95, 97, 98,
130, 156

Plough Pose, 17

power, 31

prana, 6, 13, 28, 103, 104, 155–56

Pranam Mudra. *See* meditations

pranayam, 28, 56

pranic channels, 29

pranic force, 11

pranic power, 168

prayer, 71

pregnancy, 17

prosperity, 140, 144

protection, 80

purification, 59, 168

R

rectum, 13

regeneration, 56

rejuvenation, 45

relaxation, 24, 34, 36–37, 38, 41, 105, 107–8

Rock Pose, 61, 159

Root Lock, 13, 17

S

sadhana, 50

Sanskrit, 7

Sat Kriya. *See* meditations

Sat Narayan. *See* meditations

sciatic nerve, 75

Self, 2–3

self-esteem, 145, 147

self-healing, 80, 144

self-image, 89

self-realization, 2

"Seven Steps to Prosperity," 109

sex organs, 13

sexual energy, 164

Shoulder Stand, 17, 41

Shuni Mudra, 155

Sitali Kriya. *See* Cooling Breath

sitting posture, 8

sleep, 40, 41, 42–43, 52

Sodarshan Chakra Kriya. *See* meditations

spine
    exercises for, 122

Spine Flex, 162

Spine Stretch, 46

stamina, 67

strength, 31

stress
    relief of, 38, 61, 129–30

Stretch Pose, 17, 49, 114, 117

subconscious mind
    cleansing of, 149, 156

Survasod. *See* meditations

Surya Mudra, 155

T

tattvas, 129-30

thalamus, 95

third eye, 69, 98, 110

3HO Foundation, 17

thymus, 6

thyroid, 6, 11

Transition Stress Management, 91

V

vac siddhi, 99

Vajrasan. *See* Rock Pose

Venus Lock, 159

vitality, 31

W

Washington, George, 41

Y

Yoga
    healing effects, 15
    origins of word, 3–4
    purposes, 3
    tools of, 4

yoga kriya, 5